Introduction to
NORMAL
AUDITORY
PERCEPTION

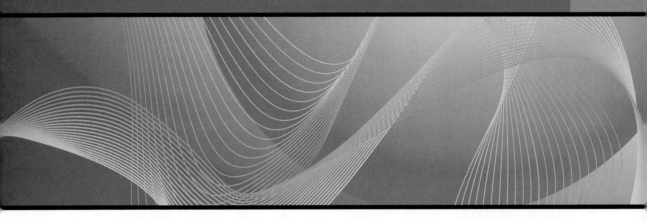

Faith Loven, Ph.D.

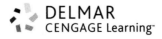

DELMAR
CENGAGE Learning

Australia • Brazil • Japan • Korea • Mexico • Singapore • Spain • United Kingdom • United States

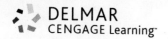

Introduction to Normal Auditory Perception
Faith Loven

Vice President, Career and Professional
Editorial: Dave Garza

Director of Learning Solutions: Matthew
Kane

Senior Acquisitions Editor: Sherry Dickinson

Managing Editor: Marah Bellegarde

Product Manager: Natalie Pashoukos

Vice President, Career and Professional
Marketing: Jennifer McAvey

Marketing Director: Wendy Mapstone

Marketing Manager: Michelle McTighe

Marketing Coordinator: Scott Chrysler

Production Director: Carolyn Miller

Production Manager: Andrew Crouth

Content Project Manager: Brooke
Greenhouse

Senior Art Director: Dave Arsenault

Technology Project Manager: Christopher
Catalina

Production Technology Analyst: Thomas
Stover

For product information and technology assistance, contact us at
Cengage Learning Customer & Sales Support, 1-800-354-9706

For permission to use material from this text or product,
submit all requests online at **www.cengage.com/permissions**
Further permissions questions can be e-mailed to
permissionrequest@cengage.com

Library of Congress Control Number: 2008938849

ISBN-13: 978-1418080778

ISBN-10: 1418080772

Delmar
5 Maxwell Drive
Clifton Park, NY 12065-2919
USA

Cengage Learning is a leading provider of customized learning solutions with office locations around the globe, including Singapore, the United Kingdom, Australia, Mexico, Brazil, and Japan. Locate your local office at:
international.cengage.com/region

Cengage Learning products are represented in Canada by
Nelson Education, Ltd.

To learn more about Delmar, visit **www.cengage.com/delmar**

Purchase any of our products at your local college store or at our preferred online store **www.ichapters.com**

Printed in Canada
1 2 3 4 5 XX 10 09 08

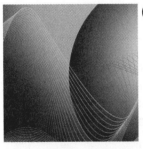

CONTENTS

PREFACE

INTRODUCTION

This textbook is designed for undergraduate students in their first course in psycho-acoustics or hearing science. It is especially geared for undergraduates in communication sciences and disorders, but it may also be useful for undergraduate majors in psychology. For students who need only an introduction to the fundamentals of normal auditory perception, this text is all-inclusive. For students who will go on to advanced academic exposure to psychoacoustics, at either the undergraduate or the graduate level, this text serves as a solid foundation of their knowledge.

AUDIENCE

This textbook takes a classical approach to psychoacoustics, presenting a basic understanding of auditory perceptions and theory by exploring the germinal research published by early researchers in hearing science. These classic investigations are explored—and, more importantly, interpreted in a way that new students can understand—to lay the foundations of modern auditory theory. The textbook starts from ground zero, taking the student through basic acoustics and seminal experiments in psychoacoustics on the role of stimulus intensity, frequency, and duration on our fundamental auditory perceptions. The basic principles of binaural listening are also covered. Students must have a basic understanding of the anatomy and physiology of the auditory system, at least in terms of the frequency-specific characteristics of the traveling wave response of the cochlea and the first-order auditory nerve fibers.

ORGANIZATION

The text is divided into five sections.

Section One covers basic acoustics as it relates to sound.

- Chapter 1 discusses simple harmonic motion, the derivation of sine waves, and pure tones. Topics include the important characteristics of simple harmonic motion, the derivation of a sine wave, Fourier analysis and synthesis, and periodic and aperiodic sounds.

- Chapter 2 explores sound transmission and sound waves, including a discussion of propagation velocity, wavelength, and sound wave motion.

- The section on acoustics concludes with Chapter 3, which covers sound measurement and the decibel (dB) scale. Discussed are the important characteristics of the decibel, the references that hearing scientists and audiologists use in the decibel scale, and a comprehensive conceptual approach to applying the decibel scale to sound measurement.

Section Two highlights the importance of stimulus intensity to auditory perception. Chapters 4–6 introduce and explore auditory sensitivity, loudness, and intensity discrimination in the normal-hearing listener.

Section Three covers the importance of stimulus frequency as a significant variable affecting auditory perception.

- Chapter 7 considers basic information concerning masking, including the effect of different kinds of maskers on detection.

- Chapter 8 introduces the concept of frequency selectivity and the critical band. Early investigations regarding the critical band theory are presented and interpreted. A basic primer on filters is also included in this chapter.

- Chapter 9 presents fundamental information on normal frequency discrimination, including a discussion of Weber's law.

- Chapter 10 completes the section with a discussion of pitch perception, which includes an extended section on classic theories of pitch perception and a modern day theory.

Section Four explores the final stimulus variable affecting auditory perception: stimulus duration.

- Chapter 11 covers the experimental evidence of stimulus duration and its effect on audibility, loudness, and discrimination.

- Chapter 12 introduces the student to auditory fatigue and adaptation.

- Concluding the text is Chapter 13, presenting a fundamental discussion of binaural listening. Included are the topics of localization, lateralization, and masking level differences.

FEATURES

- Each section includes an *introduction* that outlines the chapters included in the section and their content.

- Each chapter begins with *learning objectives* and a list of *key words*, each of which is defined in a glossary at the end of the book.

- All chapters end with a *summary of the important learning tasks* that the students should be able to do.

- Interspersed throughout the text are special highlighted sections that we call *Listen Up!* These sections either provide background tutorials to get students up to speed regarding important concepts in mathematics or physics or explain more advanced concepts.

- Finally, this text is loaded with *figures*: the graphical results of the classical studies discussed as well as conceptual drawings to help students interpret and understand basic auditory phenomena and theories.

■ SUPPLEMENT PACKAGE/ANCILLARY MATERIALS

Available for instructors is a teaching package that includes the following:

- Guided use of *Auditory Demonstrations*, a compact disk developed by A.J.M. Houtsma, T. D. Rossing, and W. M. Wagenaars and available for purchase from the Acoustical Society of America: Selected auditory demonstrations from this disk are tied to key sections of the text. Student worksheets are also included.

- Suggestions for *laboratory exercises* using a clinical audiometer and a sound booth: A handful of research questions investigating some of the major concepts of the text provide students with an in-class laboratory project experience that includes collecting and analyzing data to answer the research question at hand. All laboratory exercises require basic audiometric equipment that any university hearing clinic will have available.

- *PowerPoint slides* for lectures that include the figures in the textbook.

- A *test bank* that includes questions pertinent to the material in each chapter of the text in multiple formats, including multiple-choice, short answer longer answer, and problems.

- Two complete games of *Hearing Science Jeopardy*: Each game includes a round of regular and double Jeopardy, as well as a final round. Suggestions for making use of the Jeopardy games within the course curriculum are also included.

REVIEWERS

R. Steven Ackley
Gallaudet University
Washington, D.C.

John F. Brandt, Ph.D.
University of Kansas
Lawrence, KS

Jeffrey DiGiovanni
Ohio University
Athens, OH

Don S. Finan, Ph.D.
University of Colorado at Boulder
Boulder, CO

Marni Johnson, Au.D., CCC-A,
FAAA
University of South Dakota
Vermillion, SD

Zarin Mehta, Ph.D., CCC-A
Arizona State University
Phoenix, AZ

Joe Smaldino, Ph.D.
Illinois State University
Normal, IL

Christopher Turner, Ph.D.,
CCC-A
University of Iowa
Iowa City, IA

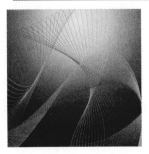

ABOUT THE AUTHOR

Faith Loven has been teaching fundamentals of hearing science and other undergraduate and graduate audiology courses at the University of Minnesota Duluth (UMD) for over 20 years. Dr. Loven earned her BS, MA, and PhD degrees from the University of Iowa and has spent her entire professional career in higher education. In addition to her courses, she has held several administrative appointments at UMD, including director of graduate studies in communication sciences and disorders and director of audiological services at the Robert F. Pierce Speech Language and Hearing Clinic on the UMD campus. She is a member of several state and national professional organizations related to audiology and higher education.

SECTION ONE

ACOUSTICS

■ CHARACTERISTICS OF THE SOUND SOURCE AND THE MEDIUM IMPORTANT TO AUDITORY PERCEPTION

The definition of acoustics is a simple one: the branch of physics concerned with the study of sound. This definition, however, is deceiving in its simplicity because the study of sound is concerned with its production, control, transmission, reception, and effects. These areas in the study of acoustics result in the many subspecialties of hearing scientists. For example, scientists primarily interested in the effects of sound on human listeners are called psychoacousticians, and their field of study is known as psychoacoustics, or hearing science.

Something known as the sound system is central to the study of acoustics and psychoacoustics. A sound system is made up of three primary components: the source, the medium, and the receiver. Each of these components focuses on a different set of concerns in the overall study of acoustics.

1. *Source:* The primary role of the sound source is to generate a vibration into the sound system. You may be familiar with common sound sources such as the speakers in electronic and digital listening devices. The human vocal folds (popularly known as vocal cords) are another everyday sound source. The common characteristic of all sound sources is that they vibrate. Much of this section of the text concerns the important parameters related to sound sources. In the first chapter of the text, we learn about vibrations and how they relate to the generation of sound. Chapter 3 shows us how the amplitude of sound sources is measured.

2. *Medium:* The medium is a collection of molecules through which the vibrations of the sound source pass. Anything can serve as a medium, as long as it is made up of molecules. So all gases, liquids, and solids can serve as the medium of a sound system. The only condition that precludes the passage of vibration is a vacuum, which by definition is a volume of space that is empty of matter. Chapter 2 of the text is concerned with some important characteristics of different media and their influence on sound waves.

3. *Receiver:* We all encounter a variety of receiver types in everyday settings. For example, the microphone in your cell phone receives the vibrations of your speech and converts them to another form of energy to serve as the sound source, in turn, for the person you are speaking with. Probably the most often used receivers in your everyday life are your ears. The human ear is our receiver for all the kinds of sounds that we need to hear. The text beyond this first section concerns the characteristics of the normal human ear as the receiver of a sound and how we perceive and interpret the information that the ear provides. Before getting into that, however, we need a basic understanding of the important characteristics related to the sound source and the sound medium, which is covered in this first section on acoustics.

The following textbooks are suggested to further your understanding of the basic principles of acoustics presented in this section.

Suggested Readings

Mullin, W. J., W. J. Gerace, J. P. Mestre, and S. L. Velleman. *Fundamentals of Sound with Applications to Speech and Hearing*, 1st ed. New York: Allyn and Bacon, Inc., 2003.

Speaks, C. E. *Introduction to Sound, Acoustics for the Hearing and Speech Sciences,* 3rd ed. Clifton Park, NY: Delmar, Cengage Learning, 1999.

Villchur, E. *Acoustics for Audiologists,* 1st ed. Clifton Park, NY: Delmar, Cengage Learning, 1999.

1

SIMPLE HARMONIC MOTION, SINE WAVES, AND PURE TONES

LEARNING OBJECTIVES

The important concepts you will learn in this chapter are:

- The definition of vibration and the types of simple vibrations.
- The definition of simple harmonic motion and its relationship to uniform angular velocity.
- The primary characteristics of graphical displays of information.
- The definition of sine waves and how they relate to simple harmonic motion.
- The important characteristics of sine waves.
- A conceptual understanding of the process of adding sine waves to form more complex vibrations.
- The common graphical representations of simple and complex vibrations.
- The definition and important characteristics of vibrations that are perceived as sound.

KEY TERMS

Abscissa
Acceleration
Amplitude
Aperiodic
Aperiodic Sounds
Cancellation
Completely Out-of-Phase
Complex Tones
Complex Wave
Continuous Spectrum
Cycle of Vibration
Dependent Variable
Direct Linear Relationship
Displacement
Envelope of the Spectrum
Equilibrium
Fourier Analysis
Fourier Synthesis
Frequency
Function
Graph
Hertz (Hz)
Independent Variable
Inverse Relationship
Line Spectrum

Linear Projection
Maximum Peak Amplitude
Noise
Ordinate
Oscillation
Parameter
Peak-to-Peak Amplitude
Period
Periodic
Periodic Sounds
Phase
Pure Tones
Repetitive Linear Motion
Simple Harmonic Motion
Sine Wave
Spectrum
Starting Phase
Summation
Transient Sound
Tuning Fork
Uniform Angular Velocity
Velocity
Vibration
Waveform
x-y Plot

OVERVIEW

In this chapter on simple harmonic motion, sine waves, and pure tones, we focus primarily on the important characteristics of the sound source. We start with a definition of vibration and learn about the fundamental variables of simple vibrations. Because the graphical representation of information is so important to our understanding of many of the experimental studies we will be exploring throughout this text, a primer concerning the fundamentals of graphs and their interpretation is also included. We explore the important characteristics of sine waves, which are the basic building blocks for many of the sounds we hear and perceive. How simple vibrations are combined to form more complex vibrations is also discussed. The chapter ends with a discussion of simple and complex vibrations and how they directly relate to sound waves. For those of you with previous academic backgrounds in acoustics, much of what is presented in this chapter is review. For those of you with limited academic backgrounds in the physical aspects of vibrations and sound sources, however, this information provides you with the basics you need to understand the remainder of the text.

VIBRATION

The primary requirement of any sound source is **vibration**. Vibration is the mechanical movement of an object, over time, around a central point or equilibrium. The term **oscillation** is also used to refer to the mechanical movement of an object.

- Vibrations can be **periodic**, meaning that the object's movement, or the oscillation, occurs regularly and consistently over time.

- Vibrations can also be **aperiodic**, that is, the oscillations do not occur in regular cycles as time moves forward.

REPETITIVE LINEAR MOTION

Perhaps the most fundamental kind of vibration is that of an object moving back and forth between two extremes repetitively over time. This type of vibration, called **repetitive linear motion**, is illustrated in Figure 1-1. At the top of this figure are three large dots. The two outer dots represent the extreme excursions of the vibration. The center dot denotes the vibration's central point, or **equilibrium**. To mimic repetitive linear motion, move your finger between the two extreme points at a constant **velocity**, or speed. Do this for a total of ten oscillations, or ten complete cycles from left to right and back again. As you try to maintain a uniform speed or velocity, think about how your finger is moving over time. Even though your finger velocity may be more or less constant, your finger's **acceleration**, or how its velocity is changing over time, is not. Within a single oscillation, starting from the left-hand dot, your finger's acceleration increases until it reaches the equilibrium

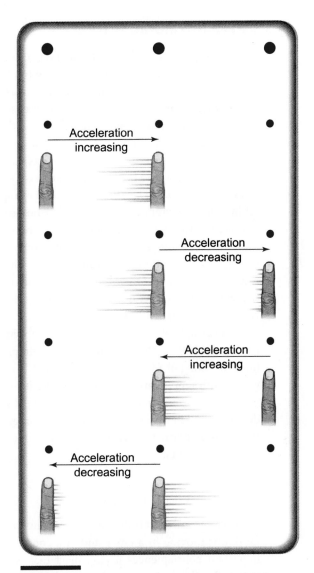

FIGURE 1-1 Repetitive Linear Motion: Let your fingers do the walking to illustrate the basic concepts of this type of motion.

point, or the midpoint. From there, the acceleration must decrease, so that you can stop at the right-hand dot. At this point, your finger's acceleration and velocity equal zero. As your finger starts to move in the opposite direction, toward the left-hand dot, acceleration increases once more in the opposite direction. Again, once the midpoint is reached, acceleration decreases, so that your finger can stop at the left-hand dot, reverse direction, and repeat the oscillation. The changes in acceleration for one complete oscillation of the vibration are also represented in Figure 1-1.

SIMPLE HARMONIC MOTION

This example of the most basic form of repetitive motion is related to another type of repetitive motion, referred to as **simple harmonic motion**. Simple harmonic motion is a fundamental vibration that forms the basic building blocks of more complex vibrations, including certain kinds of sounds. We are probably all familiar with simple, everyday objects that vibrate with simple harmonic motion. Some involve sound; some do not.

The most common examples of objects that vibrate, more or less, with simple harmonic motion are a pendulum (the one on a grandfather clock or an object tied to a string or rod) and an object on the end of a spring. Each of these objects, when set into motion, vibrates with simple harmonic motion, at least for a short period of time. In other words, the object moves between two extreme points of excursion, with constant velocity. The acceleration of the object increases and decreases during each oscillation as your finger did in Figure 1-1. In the real world, friction causes the velocity of the object to decrease over time so that it does not maintain constant velocity; however, for a relatively short period of time, its velocity changes remain fairly small.

An example of an object that moves with simple harmonic motion and that we can hear is a **tuning fork**. A tuning fork is a simple, metal, two-pronged fork with the tines consisting of a U-shaped bar of steel. When struck, the tines of the tuning fork vibrate with simple harmonic motion to produce a vibration that our ears can detect.

The vibrating tuning fork is an example of simple harmonic motion, which is defined as the linear projection of uniform angular velocity. What do we mean by the phrases "linear projection" and "uniform angular velocity"? Let's explain the second phrase first.

Uniform Angular Velocity

Uniform angular velocity means that an object moving with simple harmonic motion is moving in a circle and at a constant speed. Figure 1-2 illustrates the important consequences of an object that is moving in a circle with constant speed. This figure shows an object (a dot) moving in a circle, clockwise, with uniform velocity. The object completes a full turn around the circle in 1 s. We also know that, by traveling completely around a circle, the object travels 360°. Because the object is moving with constant speed, the object moves the same distance, in degrees per unit of time, no matter where on the circle it happens to be.

Figure 1-2 also shows four points on the circle where we have stopped time to take note of how many degrees the object has traveled and how much time has elapsed.

1. *Point 1:* Notice when and where time begins for our object. We mark this spot on the circle as 0° and 0 s.

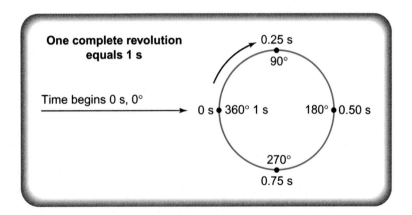

FIGURE 1-2 **Uniform Angular Velocity.**

2. *Point 2:* We allow 0.25 s to elapse, stop time, and find that our object has traveled 90° or a quarter of the circumference of the circle.

3. *Point 3:* Time starts again and we allow another 0.25 s to elapse. Then we stop time once again and see that the object has traveled another 90° around the circle. The position of the object is now 180° from the starting position, and a total of 0.5 s has elapsed since the cycle began.

4. *Point 4:* We allow another 0.25 s to elapse and stop time, and, not surprisingly, the object has traveled yet another 90° around the circle. We mark this spot as 270° from the starting position, three-quarters of the way around the circle. It has taken the object 0.75 s to make it to this point on the circumference of the circle.

For the object to move full circle, another 0.25 s must elapse. Now the object is in exactly the same position as when the cycle began (0s, 0°); to indicate that the object has completed one trip around the circle, we rename this position 360° and 1 s.

The example in Figure 1-2 shows that, because the object is moving with constant speed, 0.25 s is the same as 90° of rotation. Where the object is on the circumference of the circle when time begins doesn't matter; for every 0.25 s of elapsed time, the object moves 90° clockwise. The velocity is uniform. This would not be the case if the object moved faster, say, at the top or bottom of the circle. In other words, if the object moved with greater velocity at the top of the circle, compared to other points along the circumference of the circle, then the object would travel more than 90° in 0.25 s. For simple harmonic motion, *uniform* angular velocity is a requisite.

Linear Projection

Recall that the other part of the definition of simple harmonic motion is linear projection. **Linear projection** simply means that we are going to represent,

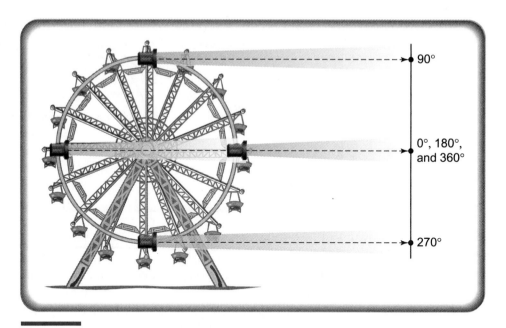

FIGURE 1-3 Linear Projection of Uniform Angular Velocity Using a Ferris Wheel.

or project, the movement of the object around the circle in a one-dimensional view. Figure 1-3 provides an example of how we might show this. In the figure, we have replaced the dot in Figure 1-2 with you. You are riding a Ferris wheel. It's night, and you have a flashlight. Straight ahead, perpendicular to the Ferris wheel is a wall. Your job is to keep your flashlight beam pointed at the wall while the Ferris wheel is turning. As you might have guessed, the Ferris wheel rotates with constant velocity.

How does the beam of light move on the wall as you make one round trip on the Ferris wheel? Figure 1-3 identifies the position of the beam of light on the wall for five selected positions during your one-cycle trip.

- When time begins (at 0 s, 0°), the beam from your flashlight is projected on the wall at 0°. From this point, time begins, and so does the ride.

- You make it to the top of the Ferris wheel, all the while keeping your flashlight beam directed at the wall in front of you. We stop the Ferris wheel and notice that your flashlight beam has moved higher up on the wall and is marked as 90°; this is its position after you have traveled 90° around the wheel. The ride is allowed to start again, and you turn another 90°.

- We stop the Ferris wheel again and take note of the position of your flashlight beam. The beam is exactly where it was when this whole process started (0 s, 0°)! How can this be? You've traveled 180° around the Ferris wheel and your light beam is back to where it started. In the three-dimensional movement of the Ferris wheel, you indeed are in a different place than where you were when time began. However, your motion is limited to just a one-dimensional display (up-down) when represented as the linear projection of your flashlight beam. So, even though at the 180° position you are closer to the wall than you were at 0°, this change isn't included in the one-dimensional representation of your movement. All that's represented is how high you are. When you are at 0° and at 180°, you're the same height off the ground.

- The wheel starts up again and you turn another 90°, stopping at the bottom. The flashlight beam's position on the wall is marked accordingly as 270°, because you are now three-quarters of the way around the Ferris wheel.

- The ride starts up again, we allow another 90° of rotation, and you're back to your starting point. The light beam is now at the same location it was at 0° and 180°. In Figure 1-3, we mark this position as 360°.

Now imagine we allow the Ferris wheel to keep rotating without stopping (again, with constant velocity). Using Figure 1-3, allow your finger to trace the continuous motion of the flashlight beam on the wall. You may notice after several revolutions of the wheel that your finger is moving in exactly the same way as was demonstrated in Figure 1-1. In other words, your finger is vibrating or oscillating between two extremes, the top and bottom of the Ferris wheel, around a central point or equilibrium.

Watching the flashlight beam move up and down a wall, although fascinating, doesn't provide us with a lot of information. Let's introduce the variable of time and see how the height of the beam of light varies as a function of time. Refer to Figure 1-4. On the left side of the figure is the Ferris wheel. Imagine the wheel is turning clockwise at a constant velocity of one complete revolution every 10 s of elapsed time. The circumference of the wheel is marked for every 45° of rotation. Because the Ferris wheel makes one complete revolution every 10 s and, more importantly, because the angular velocity of the wheel is uniform, we can assume that it will take the rider 1.25 s to travel 45° of rotation at any point on the Ferris wheel. On the right side of the figure is a plot, or **graph** (the tracing of the beam of light on the wall). The amplitude (height) of the beam of light on the wall is plotted on the **ordinate**, or y-axis of the graph. The elapsed time, from when the Ferris wheel begins to turn, is plotted on the **abscissa**, or x-axis. The function represented plots the amplitude of the beam of light at each 45° of rotation, or every 1.25 s of elapsed time. The resulting graph is the **waveform** of your motion on the Ferris wheel, or simple harmonic motion. When the amplitude of an object, vibrating with simple harmonic motion, is displayed as a function of time, the resulting function or graph is referred to as the waveform of a **sine wave**.

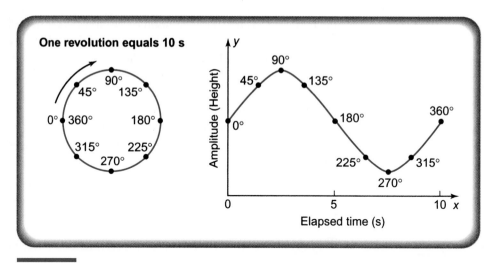

FIGURE 1-4 **Derivation of the Sine Wave.**

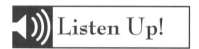

UNDERSTANDING GRAPHS

The results of a scientific experiment are often represented in graphs. Graphical representation of the relationship between two or more experimental variables makes it easier for the reader to visualize how variables are related and for the researchers to summarize their experimental results. Throughout this textbook, we will be examining and interpreting results from many different experiments related to our auditory perceptions. As a result, you need to have a basic understanding of how the variables of an experimental study are typically presented.

Most experimental studies related to hearing science involve how an **independent variable** of interest to the scientist affects a **dependent variable**. In the design of experiments, the independent variable is the one that is deliberately manipulated by the experimenter to invoke a change in the subject's response. The dependent variable is a measure of the observed response from the subject due to exposure to the independent variable. Not in all cases, but usually in hearing science experiments, the independent variable is an acoustic parameter of a stimulus (e.g., duration, frequency, intensity), and the dependent variable is some measure of listeners' auditory perception related to the sounds they hear. Remember that the levels of the independent variable presented to the subject or listener are under the *experimenter's* control. The levels of the dependent variable consist of the *listeners'* responses or perceptions of the sound. The dependent variable reflects the data that the subjects provide and that the experimenter collects.

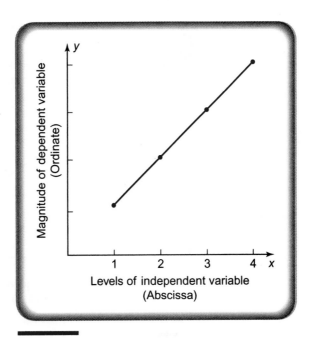

FIGURE 1-1 Generic x-y Plot with One Independent Variable.

Almost all of the experimental data presented throughout this textbook are in terms of an **x-y plot**. This type of plot is a very common way for scientists to graphically represent the results of their studies. An example of an *x-y* plot is shown in Figure 1-5.

- In the figure, four levels of a single independent variable are represented on the horizontal *x*-axis (referred to as the abscissa). For example, the independent variable, under the control of the experimenter, might be different levels of intensity of a particular sound presented to a listener.

- The listener's responses are represented on the vertical *y*-axis (referred to as the ordinate). In most of the experimental *x-y* plots that we will be looking at, the responses from listeners relate in some way to their auditory perception of the sounds presented to them. The dependent variable, the data recorded by the experimenter in response to the listener's perceptions, is always plotted on the *y*-axis.

In Figure 1-5, we see evidence of a **direct linear relationship** between the levels of the independent variable and the dependent variable. In other words, as the magnitude of the independent variable (under the experimenter's control) increases, so does the magnitude of the perception of that sound (the dependent variable) provided by the listener. That's the so-called direct part. Further, the increase in the dependent variable with the increase in the independent variable can be described by a straight line. That's the linear part. The single line represented in Figure 1-5, illustrating the relationship between the dependent and independent variables, is referred to as the **function**, which in this example is direct and linear.

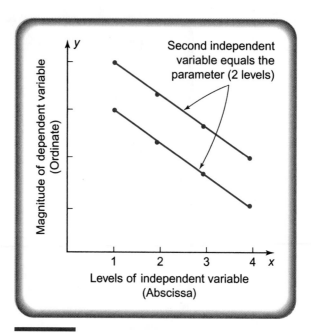

FIGURE 1-6 Generic *x-y* Plot with Two Independent
Variables.

Often experimenters explore the effect of two independent variables simultaneously on a single dependent variable. An illustration of the *x-y* plot of a more complex experimental study, involving two independent variables, is shown in Figure 1-6. In this example, the four different levels of the first independent variable are plotted on the abscissa; the dependent variable, as always, is plotted on the ordinate. The two different levels of the second independent variable are represented by the two functions (or lines) on the graph. Each function reflects a different level of the second independent variable presented by the experimenter.

When illustrated in this way, the second independent variable is referred to as the **parameter** of the graph. In Figure 1-6, we see that both functions, representing two levels of the second independent variable (the parameter), are indirectly and linearly related to the dependent variable. In other words, as the magnitude of the first independent variable (one of two variables under the experimenter's control) increases, the magnitude of the dependent variable (provided by the listener) decreases. This relationship between the first independent variable, plotted on the abscissa of the graph, appears to be also the case for each level of the second independent variable, the parameter.

When a dependent variable is indirectly related to an independent variable, we refer to this as an **inverse relationship**. It means that the magnitudes of the variables change in opposite directions; as one increases, the other decreases. In the *x-y* plot shown in Figure 1-6, the two functions are parallel. Therefore:

• The inverse relationship between the dependent variable and the first independent variable is not dependent on the level of the second dependent variable.

- The indirect linear relationship between the first independent variable and the dependent variable is the same, regardless of the level of the second independent variable.

What is different, depending on the level of the second independent variable, is the overall magnitude of the dependent variable.

- One function, representing one level of the second independent variable, consistently results in *higher* magnitudes of the dependent variable.

- The second function, representing a different level of the second independent variable, consistently results in *lower* magnitudes of the dependent variable.

■ SINE WAVES

Figure 1-7 illustrates the waveform of a generic sine wave. Notice that **displacement**, which is similar to amplitude, is plotted on the ordinate of the graph and that it is represented as a positive maximum and negative maximum, centered on a point of equilibrium (0). This is because the vibratory motion of an object moving with simple harmonic motion is characterized by movement between two extreme points of excursion around a central point.

The unit of displacement (on the ordinate) can be anything related to the magnitude of the vibrating object. Some common examples are units of distance (meters, feet, inches, or centimeters) and units of energy (voltage or sound

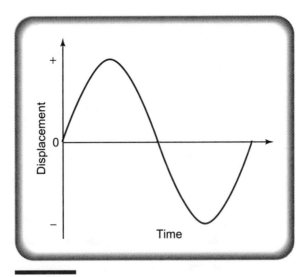

FIGURE 1-7 **Waveform Display of a Generic Sine Wave.**

pressure level). In the waveform display, time is *always* the variable plotted on the abscissa. The units used to express the measurement of time may vary (days, hours, minutes, seconds, milliseconds), but they always reflect elapsed time or duration. Whenever the waveform of a vibration looks like this, it is referred to as a sine wave and illustrates simple harmonic motion of the vibratory object.

IMPORTANT CHARACTERISTICS OF SINE WAVES

Simple harmonic motion may be expressed mathematically. Though the mathematical expression of a sine wave is beyond the scope of this text, it is mentioned because it involves the three primary parameters, or characteristics, of the sine wave:

1. Amplitude.

2. Period (or frequency).

3. Phase.

Once each of these three characteristics is known, the sine wave can be displayed graphically as a waveform or mathematically as an equation.

Amplitude of a Sine Wave

Amplitude represents some measure of the magnitude or strength of the vibration over time. Figure 1-8 illustrates the waveform of two sine waves, A and B, whose

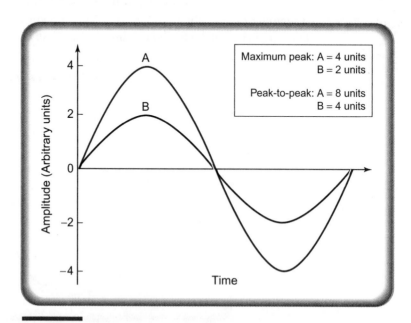

FIGURE 1-8 Two Sine Waves of Different Amplitudes: Two common methods of expressing the amplitude of a sine wave are illustrated.

amplitudes differ. (Recall that the displacement, or amplitude, of a sine wave is displayed on the *y*-axis of the waveform plot.) Clearly, waveform A possesses a larger amplitude than waveform B.

The amplitude of a sine wave may be expressed in a couple of ways.

1. The **maximum peak amplitude** represents the maximum number of amplitude units the sine wave possesses in either the positive or negative direction. In other words, it is the magnitude of the excursion from equilibrium. In Figure 1-8, sine wave A has a maximum peak amplitude of 4 units; sine wave B has a maximum peak amplitude of 2 units.

2. Another way to express the magnitude of a sine wave is to calculate the **peak-to-peak amplitude.** Using this method, the overall amplitude of the sine wave, in both the positive and negative directions, is found. Peak-to-peak amplitude takes into account the full magnitude of excursion around the central point. From Figure 1-8, the peak-to-peak amplitude of sine wave A is 8 units, and the peak-to-peak amplitude of sine wave B is 4 units.

In our Ferris wheel illustration of simple harmonic motion, the amplitude of the sine wave is determined by the height of the wheel. Figure 1-9 illustrates this relationship. On the left side of the figure are two Ferris wheels, A and B. Notice that Ferris wheel B is much smaller in diameter than Ferris wheel A. The right side of the figure shows the linear projection of the uniform angular motion of each wheel as a function of time. Clearly, the amplitude of the waveform from Ferris wheel A is larger than the amplitude from Ferris wheel B.

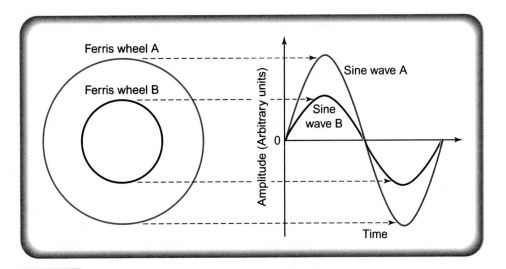

FIGURE 1-9 **Relationship Between the Amplitude of a Sine Wave and the Height of a Ferris Wheel.**

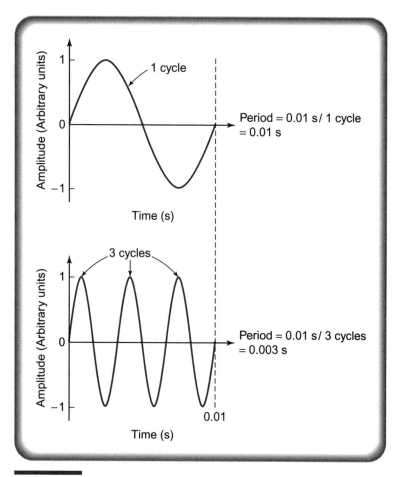

FIGURE 1-10 Determining the Period of Two Sine Waves.

Period of a Sine Wave

The **period** of a sine wave is determined by the length of time it takes the oscillating object to complete one **cycle of vibration**. From our Ferris wheel example, the period is determined by the length of time it takes you to make one complete trip (360°) around the ride. This, of course, depends on the speed of rotation, or the angular velocity, of the wheel. Period is always expressed in a unit of time.

Figure 1-10 illustrates the waveforms of two different sine waves. Both sine waves have equal amplitudes (1 unit) but different periods. The period of a sine wave is always expressed as a unit of time, and you may find it helpful to think of the unit of period as time/number of cycles. In other words, in a given length of time, how many cycles does the sine wave complete? In Figure 1-10:

- The top sine wave completes one cycle in 0.01 s. The period is calculated using the expression 0.01 s/1 cycle. This yields a period of 0.01 s.

- The bottom sine wave completes three cycles in 0.01 s. Its period is determined by the expression 0.01 s/3 cycles, or 0.003 s.

In comparing the two sine waves illustrated in Figure 1-10, the top sine wave has the *longer* period and the bottom waveform has the *shorter* period.

Frequency of a Sine Wave

The **frequency** of a sine wave shares a special relationship with its period. Specifically, the frequency is always the inverse of the period. When two variables, like period and frequency, are inversely related, we invert the numerator and denominator of one expression to find the other.

Given that the period of a sine wave is expressed as the unit of time/number of cycles, to find frequency, we invert the unit, making it the number of cycles/time. So frequency is determined by the number of cycles completed by the sine wave for each unit of time, usually 1 s.

Figure 1-11 provides an illustration, which shows the plotted waveforms of the same two sine waves from Figure 1-10. Now we calculate the frequency of each sine wave.

- The top sine wave completes one cycle in 0.01 s, or 1 cycle/0.01 s.
  If we divide 1 by 0.01 (i.e., take the inverse of 0.01), we come up with
  100 cycles/s. So the frequency of the top sine wave is 100 cycles/s.

- The bottom sine wave completes 3 cycles in 0.01 s. Again, we divide 3 by
  0.01 (3 ÷ 0.01), and calculate a frequency of 300 cycles/s.

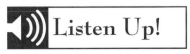 Listen Up!

FREQUENCY AND HERTZ

Scientists have unique ways of recognizing the important contributions of their peers. They often name units of measurement or important theories in honor of outstanding colleagues. Such is the case with the unit of frequency, cycles/s, which was renamed fairly recently in honor of a German scientist who discovered electromagnetism in the mid-nineteenth century. His name was Heinrich Rudolf Hertz, and in 1960 the General Conference on Weights and Measures renamed the base unit of frequency (cycles/s) to the **hertz** (**Hz**) to honor his brief but important scientific career. (Hertz died of blood poisoning at the age of 36; so his scientific career was extremely short-lived.) By 1970, the replacement of the name "hertz" for cycles/s was widespread. From now on, hertz will be used in this text as the unit of frequency; but in the back of your mind, remember that it really stands for *cycles per second*.

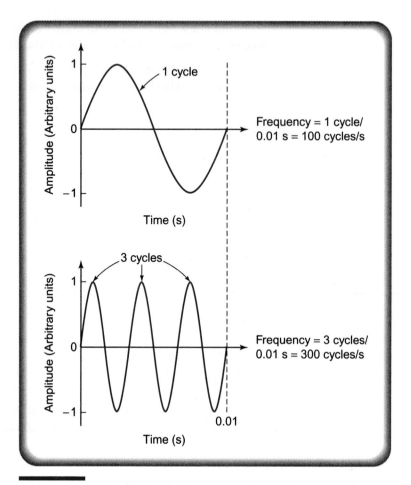

FIGURE 1-11 Determining the Frequency of Two Sine Waves.

Importance of the Inverse Relationship Between Period and Frequency

The inverse relationship between period and frequency is important for a couple of reasons.

- If the period of a sine wave is known, then the frequency of the waveform can be calculated, and vice versa. That is why frequency and period are thought of as two sides of one characteristic of a sine wave.

- The inverse relationship implies that, as the period of a sine wave increases (gets longer), its frequency decreases (gets lower). Likewise, as the period of a sine wave decreases (gets shorter), the frequency of the sine wave increases (gets higher).

As we look at the relationship between a number of variables in this text, remember that anytime two variables are inversely related, as the magnitude of one variable increases, the magnitude of the second decreases.

Phase of a Sine Wave

The third and final characteristic of a sine wave, **phase** is related to the relative position of the object at a moment of time during its oscillation and how this position compares with other sine waves. The phase of a sine wave is probably the most difficult of the three characteristics of a sine wave for beginning students of hearing science to understand. So let's return to our Ferris wheel example.

Figure 1-12 illustrates a Ferris wheel turning clockwise with uniform angular velocity. We now know several things about the wheel and its motion:

1. The linear projection of the wheel's motion yields a sine wave.

2. The size of the Ferris wheel determines the amplitude of the sine wave.

3. The speed of its rotation determines the period and frequency of the resulting sine wave.

What we need to decide is whether the point on the wheel when time begins is important. Figure 1-12 helps you answer this question. On the left side of the figure is our hypothetical Ferris wheel. Four starting points are labeled on the wheel, corresponding to the positions of the rider when time begins: 0°, 90°, 180°, and 270°. Imagine we allow the Ferris wheel to make 1½ revolutions for each of these four starting positions. The right side of the figure illustrates the waveforms of the four sine waves that result from these four different starting positions.

How do these four sine waves compare? Clearly, the amplitude and frequency (and period) of the sine waves are identical because the same Ferris wheel generated each of the waveforms. What is different among these waveforms is *the relative position of the sine wave when time begins* and throughout the 1½ cycles of the sine wave. For example, when time begins for the top waveform, labeled 0°, the sine wave is at the 0-axis crossing (the point of equilibrium) and headed up to its maximum positive excursion. When time begins, however, the second waveform, labeled 90°, is at its positive maximum value; this sine wave is at a different point of its waveform, compared to the first. These two waveforms start out 90° apart when time begins, and they will always be 90° apart at any time during the 1½ cycles of revolution. To express the difference between these two sine waves, we would say that the second sine wave is 90° out-of-phase with respect to the first. In other words, the second waveform is *lagging* the first waveform by 90°.

Now look at the third waveform, labeled 180°. When time begins, this sine wave is at the 0-axis crossing and headed down to its maximum negative excursion. This sine wave is 180° out-of-phase with the first sine wave. In other words, these two sine waves are always at opposite ends of their excursions when time

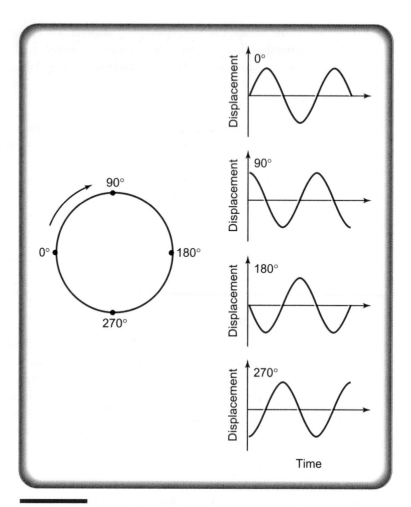

FIGURE 1-12 Four Sine Waves with Four Different Starting Phases.

begins and whenever we care to look at their amplitudes at any time during their 1½ cycles. When the first sine wave is at its most positive amplitude of excursion, the third sine wave is at its most negative. When the first sine wave is crossing the 0-axis and heading up to its positive maximum, the third sine wave is crossing the 0-axis and heading down. When two sine waves are 180° out-of-phase, we sometimes refer to them as being **completely out-of-phase.**

Now compare the third waveform (180°) with the second (90°). What is the phase relationship between the two? The third sine wave is lagging the second by 90°. It is 90° out-of-phase relative to the second waveform.

In addition to being very useful for comparing sine waves, phase is also helpful in specifying the relative position of the sine wave when time begins, a position we

TABLE 1-1 **Phase Differences Between Two Sine Waves as a Function of Starting Phase.**

		STARTING PHASE OF SECOND SINE WAVE			
		0°	90°	180°	270°
STARTING PHASE OF FIRST SINE WAVE	0°	0° phase difference	90° phase difference	180° phase difference	270° phase difference
	90°	90° phase difference	0° phase difference	90° phase difference	180° phase difference
	180°	180° phase difference	90° phase difference	0° phase difference	90° phase difference
	270°	270° phase difference	180° phase difference	90° phase difference	0° phase difference

sometimes refer to as the **starting phase**. As you might have already concluded, the top of the circle is, by convention, 90°, and the bottom of the circle is 270°. The left side of the circle is 0°, and 180° is on the right side. Table 1-1 presents the phase differences between two sine waves with identical frequency and amplitude, depending on their starting phase, or their relative positions, when time begins.

ADDING SINE WAVES

As already stated, sine waves are the building blocks of more complex vibrations. Now that we understand the basic characteristics of sine waves, we can see how different sine waves can be added together to produce more complex motions.

How do we add sine waves and determine the characteristics of the resulting combined wave? Because sine waves can be described mathematically, we can combine two or more of them by performing a mathematical operation. The resulting complex wave takes the form of another mathematical expression. Clearly, this process is beyond the scope of this text; so we take a more conceptual approach.

Figure 1-13 illustrates the waveforms of two component sine waves combined to produce a more complex wave. One sine wave has a frequency of 500 Hz, the other a frequency of 100 Hz. The 100-Hz sine wave has a larger amplitude than the 500-Hz sine wave, and both have a starting phase of 0°. The third waveform is the complex vibration produced by adding the two component sine waves.

To come up with the resulting wave, the amplitude of each component sine wave is added at every point of time. When the amplitudes of the component sine waves are added at any given point in time, whether the amplitude is less than

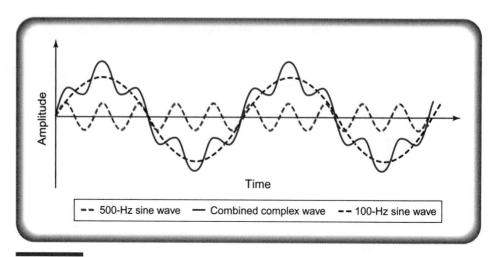

FIGURE 1-13 Waveform Display of a Complex Periodic Wave Generated from the Combination of 100-Hz and 500-Hz Sine Waves: The component sine waves are represented by the dashed functions, and the resulting complex wave is represented by the solid function.

the equilibrium (negative) or greater than the equilibrium (positive) is taken into account. For instance:

- If at a particular point in time the amplitudes of both component sine waves are below the equilibrium, the amplitude of the resulting wave *at that same point* is very negative, because we are adding two negative numbers.

- Likewise, if the amplitudes of the component sine waves, at a particular point in time, are both above the equilibrium, the amplitude of the resulting wave at that time is very positive; we are adding two positive numbers.

- Sometimes the amplitude of one component sine wave is exactly opposite the amplitude of the second sine wave at a particular instance in time. When they are added, the amplitude of the resulting vibration at that same point in time sums to zero.

You can see several instances of all three effects in Figure 1-13.

There is no limit to the number of component sine waves that can be combined using this process. Figure 1-14, for example, illustrates the waveforms of three component sine waves combined to produce a more complex vibration. The process is the same as when we were combining two sine waves. The only difference is that, with three component sine waves, we need to determine the amplitudes of all three (at a particular point in time), add them, and plot the amplitude for the combined wave. Notice that, in Figure 1-14, the three component sine waves differ in terms of their frequency, amplitude, and starting phase. There's really no limit to

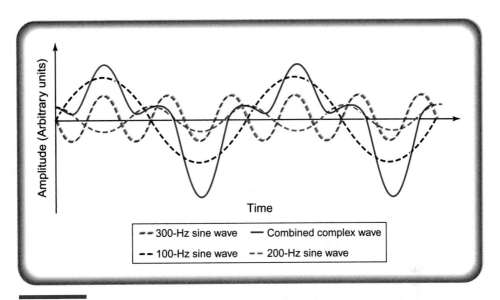

FIGURE 1-14 **Waveform Display of a Complex Periodic Wave Generated from the Combination of 100-Hz, 200-Hz, and 300-Hz Sine Waves: The component sine waves are represented by the dashed functions, and the resulting complex wave is represented by the solid function.**

the number of permutations of the amplitude, frequency, and phase characteristics of the component sine waves that can be combined.

When we combine two or more sine waves, except for some very special cases (which we explore later), the resulting vibration is no longer a sine wave. Rather, the resulting vibration is described as a **complex wave**, which is any vibration that is not a sine wave. In the examples provided in Figures 1-13 and 1-14, the waveforms of the combined disturbances are "bumpy." Sine waves, on the other hand, are symmetrical in terms of their amplitudes above and below the equilibrium. So any waveform of a vibration that is "bumpy" is a complex wave; if the waveform is smooth and symmetrical, it is a sine wave.

Also, complex waves, like those shown in Figures 1-13 and 1-14, are periodic; that is, they repeat the same changes in amplitude over time. Because the complex wave is repetitive throughout time, a period can be ascribed, just like measuring the period of a sine wave. The period of the resulting complex wave is measured as the amount of time it takes the wave to complete a single oscillation or cycle. In addition, the period of the complex wave is *always* equal to the component sine wave with the longest period or, conversely, the lowest frequency. The component sine wave that fits this criterion for both examples in Figures 1-13 and 1-14 is the 100-Hz wave. This sine wave is the one with the longest period (lowest frequency) of the combined sine waves in each example. Therefore, the period of the resulting complex wave in each example is 0.01 s.

To summarize:

- When two or more sine waves are combined, except for a few special instances, the resulting vibration is a complex periodic wave.

- The period of the complex periodic wave is equal to the period of the component sine wave with the lowest frequency of vibration.

SPECIAL CASES

There are two special cases when the combination of two or more sine waves does not result in a complex periodic wave: summation and cancellation. These special cases are illustrated in Figure 1-15.

- *Summation:* The left side of Figure 1-15 illustrates the result of adding together two sine waves of identical frequency, identical amplitude, and

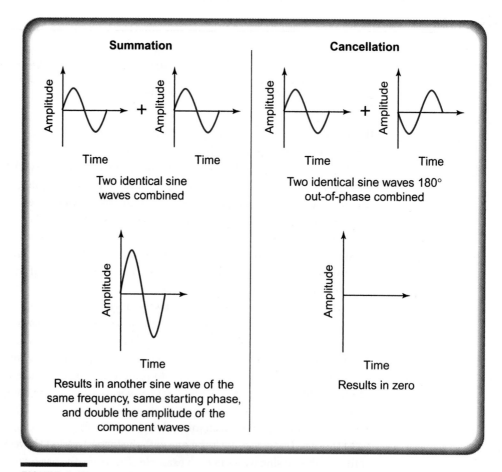

FIGURE 1-15 Illustration of Summation (left) and Cancellation of Sine Waves (right).

identical phase. The result is a sine wave of identical frequency and identical phase as the component sine waves. The amplitude of the resultant sine wave, however, is different; it is the simple sum of the amplitudes of the component sine wave. When two identical sine waves are combined, the result is summation. The only difference between the resulting wave and the component sine waves is an increase in, or summation of, the amplitude of the combined wave.

- *Cancellation:* The right side of Figure 1-15 illustrates the result of combining two sine waves of identical frequency and amplitude, but with a 180° phase difference. These two component sine waves are completely out-of-phase; when combined, they result in zero amplitude change over time— nothing. Each component wave completely cancels the vibration of the other. When you combine two identical sine waves whose phase difference is exactly 180°, complete cancellation always occurs.

FOURIER SYNTHESIS AND FOURIER ANALYSIS

The mathematical process of combining sine waves to produce more complex periodic vibrations is called **Fourier synthesis**. This mathematical algorithm is credited to Jean Baptiste Joseph Fourier, a French mathematician and physicist whose career spanned the early 1800s. (Interestingly, Fourier is also credited with discovering what is now known as the greenhouse effect, a phenomenon we hear a lot about lately, as a potential contributor to global climate change.) Fourier also demonstrated how the combination process can be performed in the reverse. In other words, given a complex periodic vibration, what are the number and characteristics of the component sine waves that result in the complex wave? Deconstructing complex vibrations to their constituent waves is called **Fourier analysis**. Fourier analysis has a broad application in a number of scientific fields other than acoustics, including statistics, signal processing, optics, and geometry.

Fourier analysis is very useful to hearing scientists because it is often helpful to know the individual components of a complex sound or vibration, especially their acoustic characteristics such as frequency, amplitude, and phase. This type of analysis gives rise to another graphical representation of complex periodic waves (in addition to the waveform), called the **spectrum**.

Figure 1-16 illustrates a complex periodic waveform along with its spectrum. The waveform at the top of Figure 1-16 is the same complex waveform shown in Figure 1-13. The bottom of the figure illustrates the spectrum of the same vibration. A spectrum plots the amplitude of the constituent sine waves as a function of their frequency. Figure 1-16 shows that the complex periodic vibration is composed of two sine waves: one at 100 Hz and the other at 500 Hz. Further, we see from the spectrum that the intensity of the 100-Hz sine wave is much larger than the intensity of the 500-Hz sine wave.

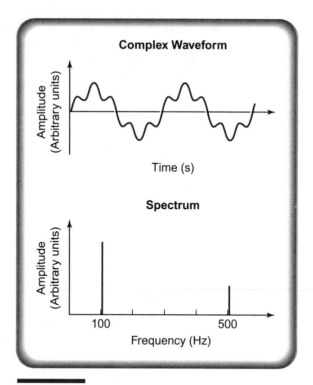

FIGURE 1-16 Display of the Waveform and the
Spectrum of a Complex Period Wave:
The complex wave in this example is
the same as that shown in Figure 1-13.

Figure 1-17 provides another illustration of a complex periodic waveform and its spectrum. The top of Figure 1-17 shows the same complex waveform represented in Figure 1-14. Below the waveform is a representation of its spectrum. From the spectral display, we can easily determine that the complex wave is the sum of three different sine waves, whose frequencies are 100 Hz, 200 Hz, and 300 Hz. Further, the 100-Hz sine wave has the largest amplitude, followed by the 300-Hz sine wave. The 200-Hz sine wave has the smallest amplitude.

Displaying complex vibrations in terms of a spectrum is much more informative and useful compared to a waveform display. When you view the waveform of a complex periodic vibration, without further information, there's not much you can say about the number of constituent sine waves that produced the vibration, let alone about their frequency and amplitude characteristics. With a spectral display, however, you can immediately determine the number of sine waves combined to produce the vibration, as well as their frequency and amplitude characteristics. Spectral displays tend to provide a more meaningful representation of complex waves, compared to waveform displays.

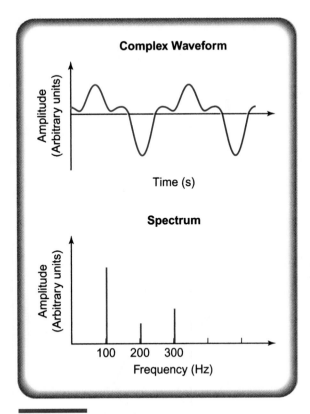

FIGURE 1-17 **Waveform and the Spectrum of a Complex Period Wave: The complex wave in this example is the same as that shown in Figure 1-4.**

■ VIBRATIONS AND SOUND

Throughout this discussion of sine waves and complex periodic vibrations, I have not used the word "sound." Not all vibrations we encounter are perceived as sound, and scientific interest in and the study of vibrations are not limited to hearing science. We conclude this chapter by defining some terms and concepts related to vibrations that give rise to the perception of sound.

PURE TONES

Periodic sound vibrations made of just a single discreet frequency or sine wave are called **pure tones**. Put another way, pure tones are sine waves we can hear. Figure 1-18 illustrates the waveform and spectrum of a 100-Hz pure tone at two different amplitudes. Notice that each spectrum of the 100-Hz pure tone is characterized by

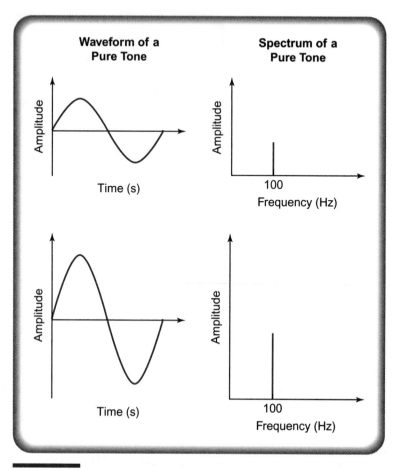

FIGURE 1-18 Waveform and Spectrum of Two Pure Tones with Different Amplitudes.

a single line at the frequency of vibration of the sine wave. A spectrum characterized by a finite number of lines is referred to as a **line spectrum**. A line spectrum simply implies that the sound produced is periodic; it repeats itself over time. If the spectrum contains only a single line, then the sound is a pure tone.

COMPLEX TONES

Complex sound vibrations, made of two or more pure tones, are called **complex tones**. The waveform and spectrum of two complex tones are illustrated in Figure 1-19. Notice that each complex tone is the combination of at least two pure tones. Therefore, the resulting vibrations are periodic yet complex because we are combining a finite number of sine waves. The spectrum of a complex tone is also referred to as a line spectrum, like the spectrum of a pure tone, because it is

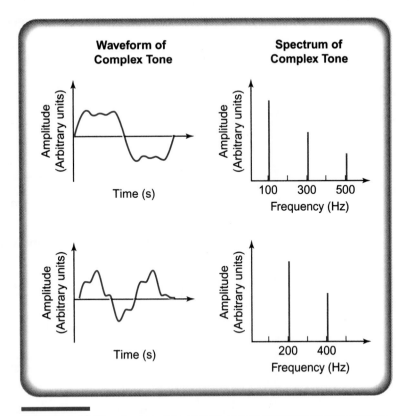

FIGURE 1-19 Waveform and Spectrum of Two Different Complex Tones.

characterized by a finite number of discreet lines at the frequencies of the constituent sine waves. Unlike the spectrum of a pure tone, however, a complex tone has more than one line because more than one pure tone is required to produce the vibration.

APERIODIC SOUNDS

Both pure tones and complex tones fall into the broad classification of **periodic sounds**, that is, sounds that repeat their waveform over time. If a sound isn't periodic, it falls into the grouping of **aperiodic sounds**, which do not repeat their waveform over time. Figure 1-20 illustrates two examples of aperiodic sounds: transient sound and noise.

Transient Sound

The top half of the figure is the waveform and spectrum of a **transient sound**, which is aperiodic because it is typically a very short-duration sound that occurs

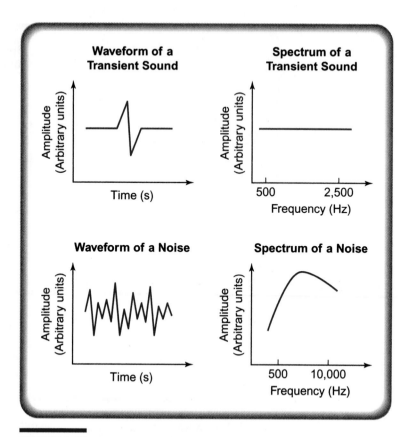

FIGURE 1-20 Waveform and Spectrum of Two Types of Aperiodic
Sound: Left—An example of a transient sound. Right—An
example of a noise.

only one time. Everyday examples of transient sounds are a gunshot, a firecracker going off, a snap of your fingers, and a single clap. Notice that the waveform of this kind of sound is characterized by a sudden increase and decrease in amplitude over a relatively short time frame.

The spectrum of the transient sound is referred to as a **continuous spectrum**, as opposed to a line spectrum. The flat line running above the frequency axis represents what is called the **envelope of the spectrum**. In a continuous spectrum, imagine an infinite number of lines (frequencies) within the envelope. Transient sounds typically have a flat, continuous spectrum with energy present throughout a relatively wide frequency range. Any kind of aperiodic sound, including transients, results in a continuous spectrum because an infinite number of frequency components make it up and they are not harmonically related.

Noise

The bottom half of Figure 1-20 represents a second kind of aperiodic sound: **noise**. Good examples of noise are the sound you hear when your radio is tuned to a frequency between two broadcasting stations or when your TV is tuned to a channel that has lost its signal. In the figure, both the waveform and the spectrum of a noise are shown. The noise waveform demonstrates a random fluctuation of amplitude as a function of time. Because the amplitude variations are random, it's not likely that the waveform repeats itself ever during the duration of the noise. For this reason, the spectrum of this noise is continuous, meaning that the frequency components making up the spectrum are not related in terms of their periods.

Again, only the envelope of the spectrum is shown. With the particular kind of noise shown in Figure 1-20, the envelope of the resulting spectrum indicates increasing spectral energy from about 500 Hz through 1,000 Hz or so. Spectral energy is relatively high between 1,000 Hz and 10,000 Hz. Above 10,000 Hz, the amplitude of the energy decreases. Notice that the frequency range of the spectral energy is relatively broad, a typical feature of aperiodic sounds.

To summarize what we have learned about the characteristics of vibrations we are able to detect:

- Sounds are broadly classified as being periodic or aperiodic.

- Periodic sounds, like pure tones and complex tones, are characterized by a line spectrum. The waveforms of these kinds of sounds repeat their variations in amplitude regularly over time.

- Aperiodic sounds either occur only one time (transient sound) or change in amplitude at random over time (noise). These sounds produce a continuous spectrum; that is, many (infinite) individual frequency components make up the sound.

▪ CHAPTER SUMMARY

We have covered many important concepts related to vibrations in general and to sound specifically. After reading and studying this chapter, you should be able to do the following:

- Define vibration and explain how it is central to the concept of the sound system.

- Define repetitive linear motion, identify the important characteristics of repetitive linear motion, and provide examples of everyday mechanical systems that vibrate with repetitive linear motion.

- Define simple harmonic motion and relate it to an object moving with uniform angular velocity.

- Provide an example of the waveform of a sine wave.

- From the waveform of a sine wave, identify and define its amplitude, period, and phase. Explain how each of these three parameters relates to the Ferris wheel.

- Explain the difference between the maximum peak amplitude and the peak-to-peak amplitude of a sine wave. Provide an example of each from the waveform of a sine wave.

- Explain and discuss the relationship between the period and frequency of a sine wave. Provide examples of calculating the frequency of a sine wave when the period is known and of calculating the period of a sine wave when the frequency is known.

- Describe the usefulness of the concept of phase when comparing two or more sine waves.

- Describe the process of combining two or more sine waves and how the period of the resulting complex wave relates to the period of the component sine waves.

- Define complex periodic waves and how they differ from sine waves.

- Describe two cases when the combination of two sine waves does not result in a complex periodic wave. Explain why these two special cases are unique.

- Define Fourier analysis and Fourier synthesis, and explain how they are related.

- Define and supply an example of a spectrum. Describe how the spectrum of a sine wave or complex wave is different from the waveform and why spectral displays are more useful to hearing scientists.

- Define a pure tone. Explain how it is related to a sine wave. Provide an example of the waveform and spectrum of a pure tone.

- Define a complex tone. Describe how complex tones are related to pure tones. Give an example of the waveform and spectrum of a complex tone.

- Define aperiodic sounds and identify the important ways they are different from periodic sounds. Provide a waveform example and a spectrum example of two types of aperiodic sounds.

2

SOUND TRANSMISSION AND SOUND WAVES

LEARNING OBJECTIVES

The important concepts you will learn in this chapter are:

- The importance of the medium's physical characteristics in the transmission of sound waves.
- How the vibrations of a sound source are propagated through a medium.
- The process of receiving sound vibrations.
- The fundamentals of sound transmission and the characteristics of sound waves.
- How sound waves are fundamentally different from other kinds of waves in our physical environment.

KEY TERMS

Atmospheric Pressure
Condensation
Density
Helium
Longitudinal Wave Motion
Medium

Pressure
Propagation Velocity
Rarefaction
Transverse Wave Motion
Tuning Fork
Wavelength

■ OVERVIEW

Having explored important properties related to the source of a sound system—vibrations—we turn our attention to the characteristics of the medium and its effect on the transmission of vibrations. In this chapter, we review how sound source vibrations pass through a medium to create sound waves. We also define some important characteristics of sound waves and discuss how they are different from other kinds of waves we encounter in everyday settings. A medium's physical properties have important effects on how vibrations are ultimately perceived, so we review those as well.

■ SOUND TRANSMISSION

The **medium** (the collection of molecules through which the vibrations of the sound source pass) plays an important role in the transmission of a sound wave. In the sound system, the medium is the conduit for the sound wave. It allows the disturbance from the sound source to travel relatively large distances to reach a receiver. Perhaps the most important job of the medium is to recreate the vibrations of the sound source so that, by the time they reach the receiver, the vibrations' critical physical parameters arrive intact.

THE SOURCE

The simplest of sound sources is the **tuning fork,** a metal, two-pronged fork with the tines formed from a U-shaped bar of steel. When struck, the tines vibrate with simple harmonic motion. In other words, the waveform of the tines' vibration is a sine wave, which we perceive as a pure tone. Figure 2-1 illustrates the vibration of a tuning fork. The figure provides a schematic of the tines' various positions relative to simple harmonic motion and the waveform of the sine wave it generates. When time begins, the tines of the tuning fork are at rest, that is, in their equilibrium position. In terms of simple harmonic motion, this is represented as 0° on the waveform (marked by the small dot).

- Time begins, the tuning fork is set into vibration, and we allow a quarter of the period of the pure tone (denoted as T) to elapse. Recall that one-quarter of the period T is equivalent to 90° rotation and reflects the positive maximum amplitude of the resulting waveform. At this point, the tines of the tuning fork are as far apart as they will go.

- Allowing time to continue for another one-quarter T, we see that the tines of the tuning fork are back to their rest position, or equilibrium. At this point, a total of one-half T has elapsed, corresponding to 180° rotation, as illustrated by the position of the dot at the point of equilibrium on the waveform.

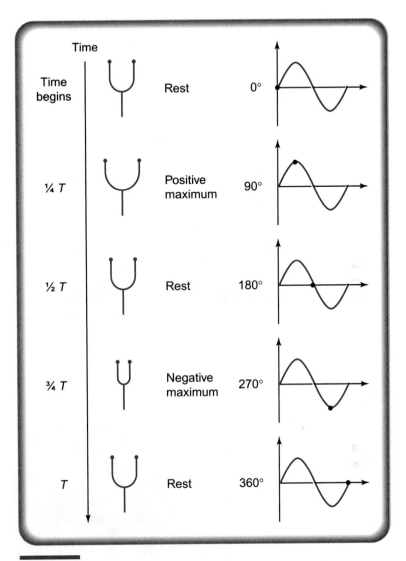

- If we allow another quarter of T to elapse, three-quarters of the period would have gone by since time began, and we see that the tines of the tuning fork are now as close together as they will ever be. This position represents 270° rotation and corresponds to the maximum negative amplitude of the wave form.

- Completing the cycle of vibration, another one-quarter of T elapses, and the tines of the tuning fork return to their rest position. This corresponds to 360° rotation and to the point on the waveform of the sine wave corresponding to equilibrium. At this point, the cycle of vibration repeats and continues until the movement of the tines are slowed, and ultimately stopped by the force of friction.

THE MEDIUM

With these characteristics of the vibration of the tuning fork in mind, imagine that the fork is placed in a medium (i.e., anything composed of molecules). How closely packed together the medium's molecules are determines its **density**. If the medium is a solid, the density is high. If the medium is a gas, the density is relatively low. If the medium is a liquid, the density is somewhere between that of a solid and a gas. Because we typically perceive sound waves in air, let's assume the medium in this example is air.

Figure 2-2 illustrates the effect of a continuously vibrating tuning fork on the distribution of the molecules in our gas medium—air. Surrounding the sound source—the tuning fork in the center of the figure—are concentric circles of varying regions of molecular density. Around the sound source are regions where the density of the molecules of the medium is higher than normal and regions where the density of the molecules is lower than normal.

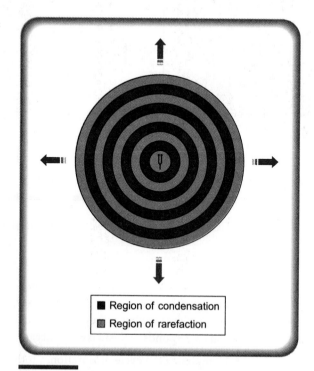

FIGURE 2-2 Propagation of the Disturbance from a Tuning Fork Through a Medium.

- The concentric circles around the sound source, corresponding to regions of higher molecular density, are referred to as regions of **condensation**. In the regions of condensation, the tuning fork tines are far apart, and the amplitude of the waveform of the sine wave is positive with respect to the equilibrium point. (The air pressure is higher than atmospheric pressure.)

- In contrast, the concentric circles corresponding to regions of lower molecular density are called regions of **rarefaction**. In the regions of rarefaction, the tines are close together, and the amplitude of the waveform of the sine wave is negative with respect to equilibrium. (The air pressure is lower than atmospheric pressure.)

Notice that the regions of condensation and rarefaction emanate outward from the tuning fork in all directions. As long as the waves of condensation and rarefaction don't encounter a boundary, like the wall of an enclosure, the concentric circles surrounding the source will continue to grow, pushing the disturbance to distances farther away from the sound source. Keep in mind that a two-dimensional display of the sound source's disturbance throughout the medium is limited. In reality, the alternating waves of condensation and rarefaction emanate spherically from the source, in all directions.

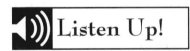 Listen Up!

CHANGES IN DENSITY AND SOUND WAVES

Changes in medium density are quite large as it moves from a gas, to a liquid, to a solid state. For example, the density of air, depending on temperature, ranges from 1.16 kg/m^3 to 1.34 kg/m^3 at 1 atm (atmosphere). The density of water, however, ranges from 958 kg/m^3 to 999 kg/m^3, again depending on temperature—a nearly 900-fold increase in density as the medium changes from a gas to a liquid. On the other hand, the relative changes in the density of a gaseous medium surrounding a sound source, like that illustrated in Figure 2-2, are very, very small. In fact, the changes in the distribution of the air molecules surrounding a vibrating source are usually measured not in terms of density, but in terms of a change in **pressure**, which is the force per unit area applied on a surface. The pressure from the air surrounding us—atmospheric pressure—is simply the weight of air at any point on earth. Although the density of air changes ever so slightly with atmospheric pressure, the small changes in atmospheric pressure that occur within the regions of condensation and rarefaction resulting from the vibration of a sound source aren't enough to change the density of air significantly. The regions of condensation are characterized by infinitesimally small increases in the density of the medium, compared to equilibrium. Because they are so small, the regions are commonly measured as a change in pressure rather than as a change in density.

Despite all that, density is usually an easier concept for beginning students to grasp than that of pressure. Just realize that they are only different measurements of our physical environment but that for our purposes they relate to the same thing.

THE RECEIVER

In our example of the sound system, the vibrating tuning fork is the sound source, and the medium is the air surrounding us. For a receiver, instead of a human ear, we place a measuring device a distance away from the source.

In Figure 2-3, the sound source is the vibrating tuning fork, at the center of the figure, and the concentric regions of condensation and rarefaction emanate from the source. A measurable distance away from the source is a measuring device, the receiver. Imagine that this device provides real-time measures of the changes in the atmospheric pressure *at this particular spot*. The tuning fork continues to vibrate, with waves of condensation and rarefaction washing over the meter. Keeping track of the changes in air pressure as time continues, we record the magnitude of the changes.

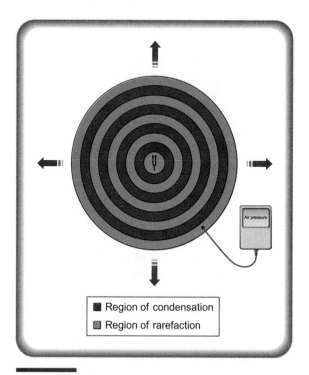

FIGURE 2-3 Measurement of Changes of Air Pressure Brought About by a Tuning Fork.

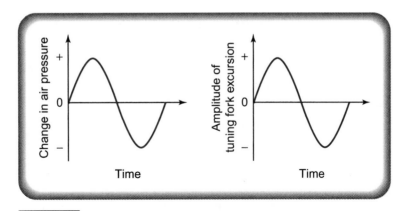

FIGURE 2-4 Comparison of the Waveform of Air Pressure Changes Resulting from the Vibration of a Tuning Fork and the Waveform of the Vibration of the Tines of a Tuning Fork.

Figure 2-4 plots our results.

- On the left side of the figure is a plot of the relative changes in atmospheric pressure as a function of time. Positive values indicate condensation (when the air pressure is higher than atmospheric pressure), and negative values indicate rarefaction (when the air pressure is lower than atmospheric pressure). The equilibrium, or 0 on the *y*-axis, indicates standard ambient **atmospheric pressure**. This plot should look very familiar. It's a sine wave. In other words, the change in air pressure, as a function of time, mimics the simple harmonic motion of the sound source.

- The right side of the figure plots the vibration of the tuning fork tines, as a function of time.

Notice that both sine waves illustrated in this figure are identical in their amplitude, frequency (or period), and phase. The only difference is in the unit of the ordinate, or the *y*-axis, corresponding to amplitude. The unit of amplitude for the sound source is the relative position of the tuning fork tines. The unit of amplitude for the receiver is the change in air pressure. The medium has successfully done its job by recreating the vibration of the sound source to a form or representation that the receiver can detect.

As you can see, sound waves are merely changes in pressure that travel in waves of rarefaction and condensation and that propagate through a medium. These pressure changes, as a function of time, exactly mimic the vibrations of the sound source. The disturbances in air pressure—the waves of condensation and rarefaction—can propagate, or travel, over long distances, as long as they don't encounter a boundary. The individual molecular particles composing the medium, however, do not move far from their original position. The disturbance resulting from the sound wave can travel long distances from the source, not the individual particles themselves.

IMPORTANT CHARACTERISTICS OF SOUND TRANSMISSION AND SOUND WAVES

Some important properties of sound waves can affect how they are perceived and make them different from other types of waves encountered in everyday settings. These properties are:

- Propagation velocity.

- Wavelength.

- Sound wave motion.

PROPAGATION VELOCITY

The speed of a disturbance moving through a medium is referred to as **propagation velocity**. You might recognize this concept as the *speed of sound*. How fast the disturbance from a source moves through a medium depends solely on the properties of the medium. Propagation velocity depends on the density of the medium and is expressed in terms of units of distance per unit of time, such as feet per second. For a dense medium, like a solid, propagation velocity is relatively fast. Propagation velocity decreases as the density of the medium decreases. So, as we move a disturbance through a solid, then a liquid, and then finally a gas, the speed of the disturbance through the different media becomes progressively slower. Put another way, *propagation velocity and medium density are directly related.*

Here is an example that may help you remember this relationship. In the early days of television, a popular program was one about the adventures of the Lone Ranger, a cowboy hero in the days of the Old West who, along with his Native American sidekick Tonto and his horse Silver, fought for truth and justice. In every episode, a bad guy was ultimately captured and brought to justice through the efforts of the Lone Ranger, Silver, and Tonto. (You may have heard the Lone Ranger's cry, "Hi-Ho Silver! Away!") Many an episode found the two heroes in the middle of the desert in pursuit of the bad guy. The Lone Ranger would stop Silver, jump down from his saddle, and cup his hand to his ear. "How far are we from the bad guys, Tonto?" he would ask, "I can't hear their horses!" Tonto, far wiser than the Lone Ranger, would climb down from his horse and put his ear to the ground. After a while, he would say, "Kimosabi, they are approaching. I can hear their horses. They are just a mile away." How could Tonto tell how far away the bad guys were just by putting his ear to the ground, whereas the Lone Ranger didn't have a clue? The answer has to do with the propagation velocity of the horses' hoofbeats through the solid medium of the ground, compared to that of the same disturbance through the air. Remember that sound travels *faster* through a solid than through a gas. When Tonto put his ear to the ground, the disturbance caused by the approaching horses' hoofbeats reached him sooner than they would reach the Lone Ranger, waiting to hear them through a gas medium (the air). It appears that Tonto had a better handle on acoustics than the Lone Ranger.

The propagation velocity of a sound wave in air is approximately 1,130 ft/s (770 miles/hr). The propagation velocity of a disturbance through the ground is much faster.

WAVELENGTH

The **wavelength** of a sound wave is the distance covered by one complete cycle of disturbance within a medium. In the case of the disturbance caused by a tuning fork, the wavelength is the distance between a region of condensation to the next adjacent region of condensation or between one region of rarefaction to the next adjacent one.

The wavelength of a sound disturbance depends on the properties of the medium *and* on the sound source. So it's relatively easy to calculate the wavelength of a sound. All you need is the propagation velocity of the medium and the frequency of the sound source. The equation to calculate wavelength is

$$\lambda = \frac{s}{f}$$

where λ = wavelength, s = propagation velocity, and f = frequency.

From this formula, you can see that wavelength changes with changes in propagation velocity and frequency.

Here's an example of how the wavelength of a sound is calculated using the equation. Let's imagine a 1,000-Hz tuning fork vibrating in air. Using the equation, f = 1,000 Hz and s = 1,130 ft/s,

$$\lambda = \frac{s}{f} = \frac{1,130 \text{ ft/s}}{1,000 \text{ Hz}} = 1.13 \text{ ft}$$

Therefore, the distance between one region of condensation and the next adjacent region of condensation for the disturbance is 1.13 ft. Likewise, the distance between one region of rarefaction and the adjacent region of rarefaction is also 1.13 ft.

- *Wavelength and propagation velocity are directly related:* Notice from the wavelength equation that as a disturbance is propagated through media of different densities, the wavelength changes. For example, if a vibration of a certain frequency is passed through a solid as opposed to a gas, the wavelength is longer in the solid and shorter in the gas. Recall that a solid has a higher density than a gas, thereby causing the propagation velocity to be higher, or the vibration to move faster, compared to a gas. The change in the wavelength may ultimately bring about a change in the perception of the disturbance ultimately reaching the receiver.

- *Wavelength and frequency are inversely related:* Two sound waves, passing through the same medium, have different wavelengths depending on the frequency of the source vibration. Specifically, if the frequency of vibration is high, the wavelength is short; if the frequency of vibration is low, the wavelength is long. This should make sense to you, given the relationship between the frequency of vibration of a sound source and the frequency of air pressure changes as a function of time. In Figure 2-4, clearly, if the frequency of vibration of the sound source changes, the frequency of regions of condensation and rarefaction washing over a stationary receiver changes as well.

To help you remember the relationship between the properties of the medium and wavelength, consider this example. You are probably familiar with what happens when someone inhales a lungful of helium gas from a balloon, speaks during exhalation, and sounds like Donald Duck! **Helium** gas has a relatively low molecular weight; it has much less density than air. That's why helium-filled balloons rise unrestrained, compared to balloons filled with ordinary air. A speaker who talks after inhaling helium has momentarily changed the resonant characteristics of the vocal tract. Listeners are accustomed to receiving and perceiving voices through air. When helium momentarily replaces the air, the density characteristics of the transmitting medium are altered. Because helium is less dense than air, the propagation velocity of a disturbance is greater than it is in air. As a result, the wavelength of the sound you receive is altered, and you perceive the sound as having a higher-than-normal pitch. The acoustic dynamics are more complicated than what I have described, but you get the point: As the characteristics of the medium change, so does the propagation velocity of the disturbance, resulting in a change in our perception.

SOUND WAVE MOTION

Sound waves are different from other kinds of waves. One important difference has to do with the motion of the particles in the medium they set into vibration and with the direction of the propagation. Sound waves are an example of **longitudinal wave motion**, which means that the medium particles (the molecules) move in the same direction as the propagation of the disturbance. Other kinds of waves that exhibit longitudinal wave motion include the seismic P-waves of earthquakes or explosions.

In contrast, some waves exhibit **transverse wave motion**; that is, the medium particles move perpendicularly to the propagation of the disturbance. Examples of these types of waves are light waves and electromagnetic waves. However, perhaps water waves best illustrate transverse wave motion. Picture yourself sitting by the shore of a lake and watching a piece of driftwood floating close by. A slight wind over the lake is creating waves that move directly toward the shore. The water waves appear to be originating from somewhere out toward the horizon and to be moving in a straight line toward the shore. The piece of driftwood, however, appears to be bobbing up and down. Over time you can see that the breeze is slowly pushing the driftwood toward the shore. For short periods of observation, however, the wood moves up and down, perpendicularly to the direction of the motion of the water from the horizon to the shore. In this example of transverse wave motion, the driftwood illustrates the motion of the water particles, and the waves moving into shore show the direction of wave propagation.

Unlike water waves, sound and other types of pressure waves cause the medium particles to move in the same direction, or plane, as the direction of the disturbance. If the piece of driftwood moved with longitudinal wave motion, it would move directly toward the shore, not bob up and down in the water. The distinction between transverse and longitudinal waves is important when they strike an object in their path. Each type of wave reacts differently to the object. The difference becomes very important when you study the propagation of a sound wave in an enclosure and the effects for the sound wave as it strikes the boundaries of the enclosure. For the purposes of this text, however, it is enough to understand that not all waves we encounter in everyday life exhibit the same properties.

■ CHAPTER SUMMARY

We have covered several important concepts related to sound transmission and the medium. After reading and studying this chapter, you should be able to:

- Explain the importance of the role of the medium in the transmission of sound.

- Explain how the vibrations of a simple sound source like a tuning fork are passed to the particles of a medium.

- Provide a definition for regions of condensation and regions of rarefaction as they relate to sound waves and explain how these principles are related to the propagation of a sound disturbance through the medium.

- Define the physical concepts of density and pressure as they relate to the characteristics of a medium. Explain how they are alike.

- Describe how a receiver perceives the vibrations of a sound source as it is propagated through the medium.

- Define propagation velocity and describe how it is related to the characteristics of the medium, and provide an example of this relationship.

- Define the wavelength of a sound wave, explaining carefully how wavelength is related to the characteristics of both the sound source and the medium.

- Provide an example of how changes to the physical properties of the medium affect how the sound may be perceived by the receiver in terms of wavelength.

- Define two fundamental kinds of wave motion and provide an example of each and identify which kind of motion is characteristic of sound waves.

3

SOUND MEASUREMENT AND THE DECIBEL SCALE

<table>
<tr><td colspan="2">

LEARNING OBJECTIVES

</td><td colspan="2">

KEY TERMS

</td></tr>
<tr><td colspan="2">

The important concepts you will learn in this chapter are:

- The importance of the decibel unit and sound intensity to the study of hearing science.
- The two primary characteristics of the decibel scale.
- The difference between linear and logarithmic scales.
- The meaning of ratios.
- References commonly used for measuring sound magnitude in terms of decibels.
- Sound magnitude calculations using the intensity and pressure decibel formulas.
- A conceptual estimation of decibel values.

</td><td>

Audiometric Zero
Bel (B)
Decibel (dB)
Exponential Notation
Hearing Level (dB HL)
Intensity
Linear Scale

</td><td>

Logarithmic Scale
Pascal (Pa)
Pressure
Ratio
Sensation Level (dB SL)
Sound Pressure Level (dB SPL)

</td></tr>
</table>

■ OVERVIEW

The magnitude of sound is expressed in terms of the **decibel (dB)**. All of us have heard about the decibel, but what is it exactly? Why did scientists adopt this unit as a measure of sound magnitude? What makes it so difficult for beginning students to understand? Why is it important to understand?

The physical parameter of sound magnitude, the decibel, is not only one of the most important aspects of any signal we might encounter, but also an extremely important stimulus parameter that dictates our perceptions of sound. For example, a sound may not have sufficient amplitude for us to hear it, even though it's physically present. In addition, our perception of sounds that are loud enough for us to hear may change if their magnitude changes. Sound amplitude is an extremely important stimulus parameter, and it figures prominently in our study of normal auditory perception. We need to have a solid understanding of the concept behind its measurement scale.

■ THE DECIBEL SCALE

You must keep two important points in mind about the decibel.

> **1.** The decibel is based on a logarithmic, or log, scale.
>
> **2.** The decibel is based on a ratio.

Let's look at each concept in turn.

LOGARITHMIC SCALES

Most of us are used to dealing with numbers or scales within a relatively small range. For example, the final exam in your hearing science course may have a possible total of 100 points; so students' scores might range from 0 to 100. This isn't a large range. As another example, the distance between Duluth and Minneapolis, Minnesota, is 236 miles. Any point between these two cities is within 236 miles. Again, 0 to 236 isn't a large range. Even greater travel distances, like New York City to Los Angeles (2,446 miles) or New York City to London, England (3,565 miles), aren't unwieldy values for us to imagine.

Representing such everyday examples visually can usually be done quite well using a **linear scale** (or linear representation); that is, each incremental change at one end of the scale is equal to the same incremental change at the other end of the scale. When two variables have a linear relationship, the incremental change along the first variable is proportional to the incremental change along the second. Graphically, the relationship between the two variables is a straight line.

For example, imagine you are working at your first job. You decide to put aside $3,750.00 each year into a savings account for a down payment on your first house. Table 3-1 illustrates your savings over a five-year period (ignoring the interest on the

TABLE 3-1 **My Cumulative Savings Over Five Years.**

Year	Total Dollars Saved by the End of the Year
1	$3,750
2	$7,500
3	$11,250
4	$15,000
5	$18,750

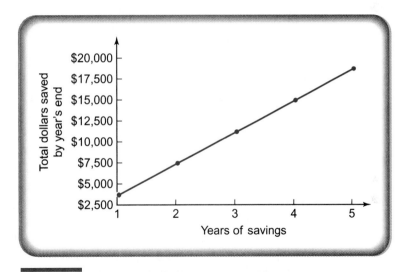

FIGURE 3-1 **My Savings History: Linear representation of the data shown in Table 3-1.**

account). Figure 3-1 displays the same information using a linear plot. In five years, you manage to save a sizable down payment of over $18,000. This linear scale easily shows your cumulative balance over the five-year period. At the end of the second year, you have a little under $8,000 in savings; by the end of year four, you have about $15,000 saved. The linear scale does a good job in illustrating your savings history over the five-year period. More importantly, this graph makes it very easy to see what your cumulative savings is at any point in time across the five years.

Most of the numbers or scales we encounter every day can be represented effectively on a linear scale. In fact, this kind of representation is so commonplace that it is hard for us to comprehend scales that are either very large or very small—like those we encounter in measuring sound intensity. Consider this fact: The range of sound pressures that the normal ear can detect is 100,000,000 to 1. If the softest sound a normal-hearing young adult listener can barely hear has a value equivalent to 1, then the loudest sound that the same listener can tolerate is 100,000,000 times larger. That's a big ratio, and unfortunately a linear representation of it won't work well.

A **logarithmic scale**, on the other hand, works very well for large numbers. Let's say you and your friend both purchase new iPods on the same day. The iPods come with 1,000 installed music downloads, and you and your friend can download an unlimited number of songs each day for 21 days for free. What a deal! The folks at Apple are interested in seeing how you and your friend take advantage of the deal; so they keep track of the total number of music downloads in your iPods at the end of each day for the 21 days. They come up with the results shown in Table 3-2, which shows that each of you started out with 1,000 songs in your iPods. Being the linear thinker that you are, you added 1,000 songs each day for a total of 21,000 songs at the end of the trial period. Your friend, however, did something remarkably different. Your friend begins the trial period with 1,000 songs and stays even with you for the first five or six days of the trial in terms of the total number of songs. After day seven, however, your friend is clearly surpassing your number of downloads each day, so that, by the end of the trial period, your friend has about 160 times more songs than you do.

The folks at Apple decide to represent your download history in a graph with a plot like the one in Figure 3-2. This plot represents your download history using a linear scale. Each axis is linear; that is, each tick on the axis is equal to the same amount. For example, on the x-axis each major tick mark is equal to one day, and on the y-axis each major tick mark is equal to 1,500 songs. This linear display of your download history is very useful to the folks at Apple. They can easily see your total number of song downloads on any given day of the trial period. For instance, if they want to see how many songs you have in your iPod by the end of day 14, the graph clearly indicates about 14,000 songs.

Your friend's download history is represented in Figure 3-3, which also uses linear representation. The x-axis scale has stayed the same: a linear representation of 21 days, with each tick mark equaling one day. However, to accommodate all the data points for the y-axis (the total number of song downloads), the range of the scale has been expanded to 3,500,000 songs. Instead of the y-axis increasing from 0 to 22,000 songs, as in the graph for your download history, it has to accommodate 3,500,000 songs to fit the range of values for your friend's downloads.

The people at Apple look at the representation of your friend's download history, and they have a problem. If they want to know, say, how many downloads your friend has accumulated by day 12, what is the value? According to Figure 3-3, the value could be anywhere between 0 and 250,000 songs. That is clearly not an accurate enough estimate for the executives at Apple. Or look at the value for

TABLE 3-2 21 Days of Cumulative Music Downloads for Me and My Best Friend.

DAY	NUMBER OF MUSIC DOWNLOADS AT THE END OF THE DAY	
	You	Your Best Friend
1	1,000	1,000
2	2,000	1,500
3	3,000	2,250
4	4,000	3,375
5	5,000	5,063
6	6,000	7,594
7	7,000	11,391
8	8,000	17,086
9	9,000	25,629
10	10,000	38,443
11	11,000	57,665
12	12,000	86,498
13	13,000	129,746
14	14,000	194,619
15	15,000	291,929
16	16,000	437,894
17	17,000	656,841
18	18,000	985,261
19	19,000	1,477,892
20	20,000	2,216,838
21	21,000	3,325,257

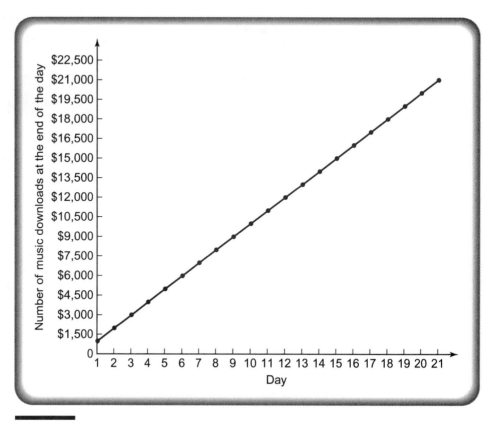

FIGURE 3-2 Your iPod Download History Using a Linear Scale: Linear representation of your music download history reported in Table 3-2.

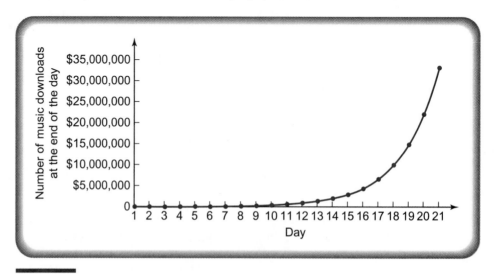

FIGURE 3-3 Your Best Friend's iPod Download History Using a Linear Scale: Linear representation of your best friend's music download history reported in Table 3-2.

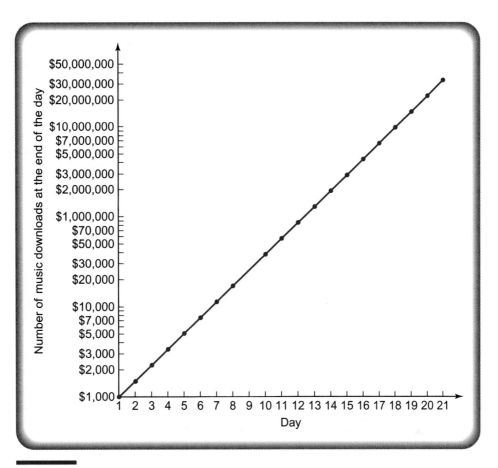

FIGURE 3-4 Your Best Friend's iPod Download History Using a Logarithmic Scale: Logarithmic representation of your best friend's music download history reported in Table 3-2.

cumulative songs after day four. According to the linear representation, the value looks like 0. We know this isn't true because both you and your friend started with 1,000 songs on day one.

A logarithmic scale allows us to represent such large numbers much more easily than a linear scale does. Figure 3-4 shows your friend's download history, with the y-axis changed from a linear to a logarithmic scale. Look at the scaling of the numbers on the y-axis. Note that:

- Each major division increases the scale tenfold. Each major division on the axis increases the value of y (the total number of song downloads) by ten times the previous amount.

- As each minor division approaches the major (tenfold) division mark, the lines get closer together (that's included for us linear thinkers).

This is a logarithmic scale.

The executives at Apple are a lot happier with the logarithmic representation. From this new display, for instance, the number of downloads that your friend has accumulated by day 12 looks like about 90,000 songs. This value is certainly more accurate than the one reflected in the linear representation. The cumulative estimate of songs after day four seems to be about 3,300 songs, a much more accurate estimate than the zero songs on the linear display.

In certain situations, thinking logarithmically provides us with a much easier and accurate display of data. Because of the range of sound pressures that the auditory system can detect is so large, a logarithmic scale is more accurate and easier to use than a linear scale.

RATIOS

The decibel scale is based on a **ratio**. For example, if two variables have a ratio of 1:2, the value of the second variable is always twice the value of the first, and, conversely, the value of the first variable is always one-half the value of the second. Likewise, if the ratio between two variables is 1:10, the second variable is always ten times the magnitude of the first, and the first variable is always one-tenth the magnitude of the second. The amplitude of a sound, expressed in decibels, represents how much larger the sound is than some reference. In the world of decibels, it's very important to specify the reference, because more than one reference is used.

■ REFERENCES USED IN THE DECIBEL SCALE

Three common references are used for the decibel scale:

1. The sound pressure level reference (dB SPL).

2. The hearing level reference (dB HL).

3. The sensation level reference (dB SL).

THE SOUND PRESSURE LEVEL REFERENCE (dB SPL)

The reference for **sound pressure level (dB SPL)** is a physical pressure that can be measured independently of a human observer. The reference is not based on any listener's perception or on any aspect of the normal auditory system. The physical pressure of the sound pressure level reference is 0.0002 dynes/cm^2, which is a very small unit of pressure. It represents a very small force (a dyne) applied over a very small area (a square centimeter). Scientists have adopted the dyne/cm^2 for the SPL reference because it represents the smallest amount of pressure detectable by a normal-hearing, young adult listener under ideal circumstances. If a sound is measured to have a pressure level equivalent to, say, 7.5 dB, the sound is 7.5 dB greater than the reference pressure of 0.0002 dynes/cm^2, or 20 μPa. It doesn't matter what kind of sound it is or whether any human is around to hear it. This is its specified pressure. The SPL reference (0.0002 dynes/cm^2) does not change with the characteristics of the signal or the receiver.

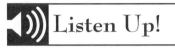 Listen Up!

UNITS OF SOUND PRESSURE

The unit of pressure relevant to sound (dynes/cm^2) represents a smaller proportion of the standard unit of pressure, newton/m^2. In 1971, the International System of Units (SI) changed the name of the newton/m^2 to the **Pascal (Pa)**, in honor of Blaise Pascal, a French mathematician, physicist, and philosopher who lived in the seventeenth century. The SI is a scientific system, formerly called the meter-kilogram-second (MKS) system, for expressing the magnitudes or quantities of important natural phenomena. The reference pressure for dB SPL (0.0002 dyne/cm^2) is equivalent to 20 μPa (micropascal). Most modern references to sound pressure level are in terms of the micropascal. For instructive purposes, however, we refer to the unit as dyne/cm^2.

THE HEARING LEVEL REFERENCE (dB HL)

The **hearing level** reference **(dB HL)** is primarily used to specify sound magnitude in the clinical setting. Almost all instruments used in clinical audiology, such as audiometers, specify sound amplitude in terms of dB HL. This reference is based on the typical sound pressure levels of pure tones that normal-hearing, young adults need just to be able to detect their presence. As we will see later, our sensitivity to pure tones depends on their frequency. In general, we are most sensitive to sounds with frequencies between 1,000 and 5,000 Hz; at these frequencies, sounds can be present at relatively low pressures and remain detectable by human listeners. Signals above or below this frequency range tend to need higher pressures for us to hear them.

In clinical situations, we are usually interested in knowing how an individual's hearing compares to what is typical for normal-hearing listeners. In other words, we might present a listener with a number of different-frequency pure tones to find the lowest sound pressure level the listener can detect them. Then we can directly compare our listener's results to what we know is the case for so-called normal hearing. The hearing level reference allows us to make this type of comparison.

The hearing level reference is based on average normal-hearing sensitivity. For example, the average lowest sound pressure level at which normal-hearing listeners can just detect the presence of a 1,000-Hz pure tone, under fairly ideal conditions, is about 7.5 dB. At 1,000 Hz, in the HL reference this amplitude is equal to 0 dB HL. In fact, we call 0 dB HL **audiometric zero** because it represents the floor of auditory sensitivity, at least as far as audiologists are concerned. Audiologists expect normal-hearing listeners to be able to just detect the presence of any sound at levels equivalent to 0 dB HL, which corresponds to the lower limit of usable hearing. So, let's say we measure the hearing of a listener whose hearing is not normal, and it is equivalent to 45 dB HL at 1,000 Hz. That person's hearing is not normal, and, further, its sensitivity departs from normal by 45 dB. This measurement gives us an idea of how much the listener's hearing departs from normal, that is, the degree of hearing loss.

A very important characteristic of the hearing level reference is that it changes depending on the kind of signal used. Because our sensitivity to sound depends on its characteristics, such as frequency, it makes sense that the reference pressure in hearing level also changes with the signal's characteristics. The reference sound pressure equivalent to 0 dB HL is different for pure tones of different frequencies, and it is different if speech is the signal used or if the signal is a noise.

Although the reference changes with the characteristic of the signal, it is *not* affected by the receiver. Anyone can be listening to the sound, the listener can be normal-hearing or not, and the receiver doesn't even have to be human. The reference pressure stays the same.

THE SENSATION LEVEL REFERENCE (dB SL)

The **sensation level (dB SL)** is a very personalized reference because it depends on the characteristics of the signal *and* the receiver. The SL reference is the lowest sound level that an individual listener is able to detect for a particular type of signal. For example, if you're able to just detect a 500-Hz tone at a sound pressure level of 15 dB, this intensity is equivalent to 0 dB SL. The reference pressure at 500 Hz for *you* is 15 dB SPL. If we were to change the frequency of the tone, the reference pressure may also change and no longer equal 15 dB SPL because your sensitivity is likely to change. Likewise, if we were to present the 500-Hz tone at 15 dB SPL to *another* listener, the reference pressure will probably change unless you both have identical sensitivity at this frequency.

▓ SOME CAVEATS REGARDING THE DECIBEL

A couple of interesting notions about the decibel need to be addressed. *Zero decibels is not the absence of sound.* In many of the everyday numerical scales we are familiar with, 0 means the absence of something. For example, if your bank account has a balance of $0, you have no money. If the gas gauge in your car registers 0 gallons, you have no gas, and you won't be going anywhere. In most cases, zero means the absence of something. Not so with the decibel scale. The phrase 0 dB does *not* mean the absence of sound. In the preceding section, 0 dB was mentioned quite a bit: 0 dB HL is equivalent to audiometric zero, and 0 dB SL corresponds to an individual's best sensitivity for a particular sound. However, the term zero simply means that the related sound pressure is equal to the reference pressure, in either sound pressure level, hearing level, or sensation level.

A familiar scale that behaves like the decibel in this regard is the temperature scale on the thermometer. Clearly, 0°F does not mean the absence of temperature. On the Fahrenheit scale, 0° simply means that the air temperature is equivalent to a reference. In fact, on some days we experience temperatures below 0°F. The coldest recorded temperature in northern Minnesota was set on February 2, 1996 at –60°F, but the record does not mean that Minnesotans had less than an absence of temperature. It simply means that the air temperature recorded on that frigid day was 60° below the reference temperature.

The same holds true for the decibel. Negative decibel values can exist in each of the reference systems. For example, most audiometers deliver sound levels as low as –10 dB HL. This level simply means that the sound is 10 dB below the reference pressure (0 dB HL or audiometric zero) for a particular signal.

Regardless of the reference, a decibel is a decibel. All decibels are created equal, whether the reference is sound pressure level, hearing level, or sensation level. The only thing that changes across the three references is the starting point, or floor, of the scale. For example, if a sound begins with a sound pressure level of 30 dB and increases to 40 dB SPL, the change in intensity is equivalent to 10 dB. If another sound begins with a hearing level of 55 dB and increases to 65 dB HL, it too represents a 10-dB increase. The change in amplitude for both sounds is the same. In other words, a 10-dB change in sound level, in terms of either sound pressure level or hearing level, represents the same *amount* of change as represented by the decibel.

■ DECIBEL COMPUTATION

You can calculate sound amplitude in decibels in two ways.

1. In terms of pressure (P):

$$20 \log \frac{P_1}{P_0}, \text{ where } P_0 = 0.0002 \text{ dynes/cm}^2$$

2. In terms of intensity (I):

$$10 \log \frac{I_1}{I_0}, \text{ where } I_0 = 10^{-16} \text{ watts/cm}^2$$

(We'll explore the difference between pressure and intensity units later.)

Look at these equations, and recall the two primary characteristics of the decibel; (1) It is based on a ratio, and (2) it is based on a logarithmic scale. Can you see in these equations:

- The ratios?

- The references?

- The logarithms?

There are several differences between these two units of sound measurement, or amplitude.

- When sound amplitude is measured in terms of **pressure**, the calculation uses the pressure ratio (P_1/P_0). The reference pressure, as already explained, is 0.0002 dynes/cm² (20 µPa), which reflects force applied to an area. Dynes/cm² is a very small unit of force applied over a very small area.

- When sound amplitude is measured in terms of **intensity**, the calculation uses the intensity ratio (I_1/I_0). The reference intensity is 10^{-16} watts/cm², which is equivalent to 0.0002 dynes/cm². Intensity is expressed as watts/cm², where a watt is a unit of work or power. Therefore, intensity is some unit of work or power applied over some unit of area.

Both references, specified in terms of either pressure or intensity, are the same. The only difference is the *physical* unit in which each is measured.

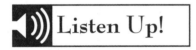 Listen Up!

WHERE DID THE DECIBEL GET ITS NAME?

The decibel (dB) is a fraction of a much larger unit of sound amplitude, the bel. The bel was invented by scientists working at the Bell Telephone Laboratory during the early days of telephone research nearly 100 years ago. The **bel (dB)** is defined as the reduction in audio level over a 1-mile length of standard telephone cable. The unit is named in honor of Alexander Graham Bell, the laboratory's founder and telecommunications pioneer. The bel is too large for practical use as a unit in the measurement of sound amplitude. The decibel (dB), which is equal to 1/10 (0.1) of a bel, is the preferred unit.

APPLYING THE EQUATIONS

Here is an example calculating the magnitude of a sound using the pressure formula:

A sound source in a room has a pressure equal to 10 dynes/cm². What's the decibel value if the reference pressure equals 0.0002 dynes/cm²?

$$20 \log 10/0.0002$$

$$20 \, (\log 50,000)$$

$$20 \, (4.699)$$

$$93.98 \text{ dB}$$

Here is an example calculating the magnitude of a sound using the intensity formula:

A sound source in a room has intensity equal to 10^{-8} watts/cm^2. What's the dB value if the reference intensity equals 10^{-16} watts/cm^2?

$$10 \log 10^{-8} \div 10^{-16}$$

$$10 \log 10^8$$

$$10\,(8)$$

$$80\,\text{dB}$$

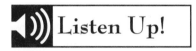 Listen Up!

A QUICK REVIEW OF EXPONENTIAL NOTATION

You may have noticed that the physical units for sound amplitude are very, very small. For this reason, these units are generally expressed in terms of **exponential notation**. You may need a quick review of this display of very small numbers.

Exponential notation is used to easily represent very large or very small numbers in terms of base 10 values. To express very large numbers using exponential notation, use the following rule:

$$10^1 = 10,\, 10^2 = 100,\, 10^3 = 1{,}000 \ldots 10^x = 1(x)$$

The exponent tells you how many zeros there are after the 1.

To express very small numbers using exponential notation, use the following rule:

$$10^{-1} = 0.1,\, 10^{-2} = 0.01,\, 10^{-3} = 0.001 \ldots 10^{-x} = 0.x \times 1$$

The exponent tells us how many places to move the decimal to the left of the 1. Notice that negative exponents represent numbers less than 1 and that positive exponents represent numbers greater than 1.

When two numbers, expressed in exponential notation, are multiplied, the exponents are *added*.

For example:

$$10^2 \times 10^5 = 10^7$$

When two numbers expressed in exponential notation, are divided, the exponents are *subtracted*.

For example:

$$10^2 \div 10^5 = 10^{-3}$$

■ CONCEPTUAL APPLICATION OF THE DECIBEL

Although the equations for the decibel are important to know, it may be more useful to take a conceptual approach to decibel calculations. The basis of this approach applies the two things we already know about the decibel: It's based on a ratio and on a logarithmic scale.

THE PRESSURE FORMULA

Let's consider the pressure formula for the decibel:

$$20 \log \frac{P_1}{P_0}$$

Remember that the ratio P_1/P_0 represents the relationship between the sound pressure of interest and the reference pressure. If the ratio of these two values is based on a factor of 10, the decibel conversion is quite simple. Consider the information in Table 3-3. Do you notice a pattern? Every time the ratio is increased tenfold, the decibel equivalent increases by 20. Another way of expressing this pattern is to count the number of 0s in the P_1/P_0 ratio and multiply by 20.

Or you can express the P_1/P_0 ratio in terms of exponential notation, as shown in Table 3-4. When the ratio is expressed this way and we take the log of that value, the log always equals the value of the exponent. The log tells us the number of zeros following the 1. After that, we simply multiply this number by 20 to get the dB equivalent. We can generalize this concept:

$$20 \log 10^x = 20(x) = \text{dB value}$$

Pressure ratios won't always be an even factor of 10, but by rounding up or rounding down, we can make a close estimate.

You have to memorize one pressure ratio: the 2:1 ratio. Whenever the ratio between P_1/P_0 equals 2:1, the decibel equivalent equals 6 dB. In other words, whenever a sound pressure is doubled, the magnitude of the sound increases by 6 dB.

TABLE 3-3 Some Common Sound Pressure Ratios and Their Decibel Equivalents.

P_1/P_0 Ratio	Decibel Equivalent (dB)
10:1	20
100:1	40
1,000:1	60
10,000:1	80

TABLE 3-4 Some Common Sound Pressure Ratios and Their Decibel Equivalents.

P_1/P_0 Ratio	Decibel Equivalent
$10^1:1$	20
$10^2:1$	40
$10^3:1$	60
$10^4:1$	80

THE INTENSITY FORMULA

When sound magnitude is measured in terms of intensity, the units are expressed in just the same way as pressure units. In Table 3-5, the I_1/I_0 ratios are expressed in factors of 10. Notice that every time the intensity ratio increases by a power of 10, the decibel equivalent increases by 10.

These ratios are expressed in terms of exponential notation in Table 3-6. Take the value of the exponent (the number of 0s following the 1) and multiply by 10 to arrive at the dB equivalent.

We can generalize this concept using the following:

$$10 \log 10^x = 10(x) = \text{dB value}$$

As was the case when working in pressure units, you have to memorize one intensity ratio: the 2:1 ratio. Whenever the ratio between I_1/I_0 equals 2:1, the decibel equivalent equals 3 dB. In other words, whenever a sound intensity is doubled, the magnitude of that sound increases by 3 dB.

TABLE 3-5 Some Common Sound Intensity Ratios and Their Decibel Equivalents.

I_1/I_0 Ratio	Decibel Equivalent
10:1	10
100:1	20
1,000:1	30
10,000:1	40

TABLE 3-6 Some Common Sound Intensity Ratios and Their Decibel Equivalents.

I_1/I_0 Ratio	Decibel Equivalent
10^1:1	10
10^2:1	20
10^3:1	30
10^4:1	40

■ EVERYDAY EXAMPLES

How can we apply what we've just learned to everyday problems involving the decibel? We can work two types of such problems using this easy approach.

1. Given the intensity or pressure ratio of one sound relative to another, what is the decibel value?

2. Given the decibel value, what is the pressure or intensity ratio?

GIVEN THE INTENSITY OR PRESSURE RATIO

The sound pressure in room A, compared to the sound pressure in room B, is 1,600,000:1. What is the magnitude of the source in room A (in decibels) with respect to room B?

Start with the pressure ratio: 1,600,000:1. Because we can easily convert pressure ratios of 2:1, 10:1, 100:1, and similar ranges, we need to factor 1,600,000 down to pressure ratios that we can convert easily:

$$2 \times 2 \times 2 \times 2 \times 100{,}000{:}1$$

All we've done is break down 1,600,000 into its factors that we can more easily convert to a decibel equivalent. Now we are ready to convert. Take each of the factors and change them to their decibel equivalent:

$$(2) \times (2) \times (2) \times (2) \times (100{,}000)$$

Once we've made the conversion, we *add* the dB equivalents

$$(6) + (6) + (6) + (6) + (100) = 124 \text{ dB}$$

This is the magnitude of the sound in room A with reference to the sound in room B: 124 dB.

That was easy. No calculators with log functions were needed. We were able to estimate the decibel value just by applying the basic characteristics of the decibel.

Let's work the same ratio using intensity. The sound intensity in room A, compared to the sound intensity in room B, is 1,600,000:1. What is the magnitude of the source in room A (in decibels) with respect to room B?

Here's the ratio: 1,600,000:1. Again, factor to intensity ratios you know:

$$2 \times 2 \times 2 \times 2 \times 100{,}000{:}1$$

Convert to decibels (remember to *add* after this step).

$$3 + 3 + 3 + 3 + 50 = 62 \text{ dB}$$

This is the magnitude of the sound in room A with reference to the sound in room B, measured in terms of intensity: 62 dB.

Notice that we worked both problems using the same ratio: 1,600,000:1. The first problem was worked in terms of pressure, the second in terms of intensity. Notice that the decibel equivalent in terms of pressure (124 dB) is twice the decibel equivalent found using intensity (62 dB). This is always the case given identical ratios of P_1/P_0 and I_1/I_0,

- The decibel equivalent of the pressure measurement is always twice the decibel equivalent of the intensity measurement.

- The decibel equivalent of the intensity measurement is always one-half the decibel equivalent of the pressure measurement.

You can see the reason for this by looking at the two formulas:

$$20 \log \frac{P_1}{P_0}, \text{ where } P_0 = 0.0002 \text{ dynes/cm}^2$$

$$10 \log \frac{I_1}{I_0}, \text{ where } I_0 = 10^{-16} \text{ watts/cm}^2$$

The log of the ratio is multiplied by either 20 (for pressure) or 10 (for intensity). Obviously, 20 is twice 10, and, conversely, 10 is one-half of 20. If the given ratios are identical in each case, the log of the ratio is the same as well. What differs is whether the result is multiplied by 10 or 20. Therefore, the decibel equivalent in terms of pressure is always twice the amount of the dB equivalent in terms of intensity.

Given the Decibel Value

Given the decibel value, what is the pressure or intensity ratio?

A sound source is emitting a pure tone at 46 dB SPL. What is the pressure ratio of the source to the reference pressure?

To solve this problem, we work backward from the exercises illustrated in the previous examples. The dB equivalent between the two sources is 46 dB SPL. Reduce 46 to decibel values that we can convert easily to the appropriate ratio. (Remember that we are dealing with pressure ratios.) Because we are still working in decibels, we need to break things down into sums rather than into factors.

$$40 + 6$$

Convert to the ratios. Working backward, 40 dB means the ratio has an exponent of 40/20, or 2, or 1 followed by 2 zeros: 100. Recall that 6 dB is equivalent to a 2:1 pressure ratio. Remember at this point, we *multiply* the factors.

$$100 \times 2$$

This represents the pressure ratio between the sound we are measuring and the reference pressure.

$$200:1$$

So the sound pressure is 200 times greater than the reference pressure.

Let's work a similar problem using the intensity reference.

A sound source is emitting a pure tone at 46 dB. What is the intensity ratio of the source to the reference intensity?

The dB equivalent between the two sources is 46 dB. Reduce 46 to decibel values we can convert easily to the appropriate ratio. (Remember that we are dealing with intensity ratios.) Because we are working in decibels, we need to break things down into sums rather than into factors.

$$40 + 3 + 3$$

Convert to the ratios. Working backward, 40 dB means that the ratio has an exponent of 40/10, or 4, or 1 followed by 4 zeros: 10,000. Recall that 3 dB is equivalent to a 2:1 intensity ratio. At this point, we multiply the factors.

$$10,000 \times 2 \times 2 = 40,000$$

This represents the intensity ratio between the sound we are measuring and the reference intensity: 40,000:1. So the sound intensity is 40,000 times greater than the reference intensity.

■ APPLYING THE DECIBEL CONCEPT TO A NEW PROBLEM

Now you should be able to estimate just about any sound's decibel value, pressure ratio, or intensity ratio. Let's look at a problem that allows you to make use of your new skills and that illustrates the unusual behavior of the decibel when two sounds are added together.

Suppose we have two sound sources. One has a sound pressure level of 86 dB SPL, and the other has a sound pressure level of 46 dB SPL. We put these two sources together in one room, turn them on, and measure the resulting sound pressure level in the room. What do you suppose the cumulative sound pressure level will be in decibels?

You may be tempted to simply add the SPL values, in decibels, from each source, coming up with a final SPL of 132 dB. Unfortunately, because the decibel is a ratio, this won't provide the correct answer. When sounds are mixed or added, their physical sound pressures combine; so we need to express each sound in terms of its pressure, not its decibels. What we need to do is:

- Reduce each decibel value to its pressure ratio.
- Add the pressures.
- Then convert the new ratio back to its dB equivalent.

Let's start by reducing each decibel equivalent to its pressure ratio. Notice that each sound magnitude is expressed in terms of sound pressure level; so we use the method corresponding to pressure units.

We reduce the decibel value of sound 1 (86 dB) to decibel values we can easily convert to pressure ratios: 80 + 6.

Now we convert to the pressure ratios. Working backward, 80 dB means that the ratio has an exponent of 80/20, or 4, or 1 followed by 4 zeros, 10,000. Recall that 6 dB is equivalent to a 2:1 pressure ratio. At this point, we multiply the factors.

$$(10{,}000) \times (2)$$

This represents the pressure ratio between the first sound and the reference pressure: 20,000:1.

Now we need to apply the same concepts to the second sound source, with an amplitude of 46 dB SPL. The decibel equivalent is reduced for the second sound to decibel values that we can easily convert to pressure ratios: 40 + 6.

Convert the ratios: 40 dB means that the ratio has an exponent of 40/20, or 2, or 1 followed by 2 zeros, or 100. Again, 6 dB is the equivalent to a 2:1 ratio.

Multiply the factors:

$$(100) \times (2)$$

This represents the pressure ratio between the first sound and the reference pressure: 200:1.

The two sounds are combined in the same room. When they are turned on, the sound pressures combine, and a new pressure ratio exists: 200 + 20,000 = 20,200:1. We need to take this new ratio and convert it to its decibel equivalent. Factor out a 2:

$$(2) \times (10{,}100)$$

Factor out 100:

$$(2) \times (100) \times (101)$$

We are left with two factors that can easily be converted to decibel equivalent, but the 101:1 ratio is not one we can easily convert. Because we need only a reasonable estimate of the new decibel value, we represent the 101:1 ratio as 100^+:1. In other words, 100:1 plus a little bit more. Now we are ready to convert to decibels.

$$(2) \times (100) \times (100^+)$$

Convert each ratio to its decibel equivalent, carrying over the little extra from the 101:1 ratio.

$$6 + 40 + 40^+$$

The final decibel value of the combined sound sources is 86^+ dB

Adding a sound source with a magnitude of 86 dB to a sound source with a smaller magnitude of 46 dB results in a combined sound magnitude of something just a little bit greater than 86 dB. In other words, the addition of the smaller magnitude sound source doesn't change things much. How can this be? When we combined the sources in terms of their sound pressure levels, we increased the overall sound pressure by only 200 dynes/cm². Compared to the original sound pressure level ratio of 20,000:1, this is a very small increase in pressure. To increase the decibel value by 6 dB, we have to double the pressure (a 2:1 ratio). Adding 200 dynes/cm² to 20,000 dynes/cm² is nowhere near doubling the pressure. So the overall increase in pressure achieved by adding the sound source with a magnitude of only 46 dB, compared to the larger sound magnitude of 86 dB, is not great.

Keep this exercise in mind when working with the decibel scale. A small increase in pressure, even though the decibel value may be significant, doesn't result in a large overall increase in pressure.

■ CHAPTER SUMMARY

We have covered many important concepts in this chapter related to sound measurement and the decibel. You should be able to do the following:

- Explain why sound magnitude and the decibel as a unit of sound magnitude are important to the field of hearing science.
- Identify and describe the two important characteristics of the decibel scale.
- Define and discuss the important characteristics of the linear and logarithmic scales.
- Explain why a logarithmic scale is necessary for measuring sound magnitude.
- Define a ratio and explain its importance to the measure of sound intensity.
- Identify the three common reference scales used for the decibel and the reference used for each one.
- Identify the two computational formulas used to calculate sound magnitude, in decibels, and explain how the two formulas differ when measuring the amplitude of a sound in terms of sound intensity and sound pressure.
- Apply each decibel formula, given either the sound intensity or the sound pressure of a sound source.
- Estimate the decibel value of two sounds, given either their intensity or pressure ratios.
- Estimate either the intensity or pressure ratio between two sounds, given their dB value.

SECTION TWO

INTENSITY

◼ INTENSITY AS AN IMPORTANT STIMULUS VARIABLE TO AUDITORY PERCEPTION

So far we have learned that sounds can be described in the physical realm in terms of intensity, frequency (or period), duration, and phase. Arguably, intensity is the most important of these acoustic parameters of sounds when it comes to influencing our perceptions. The physical amplitude of a sound has a profound influence on how we perceive it. For example, we learn that sounds must possess a minimum level of magnitude for us to sense their presence. Further, once we can "hear" a sound, altering the intensity can bring about significant changes in our perceptions of it. While the roles of the other physical parameters of a sound are important, stimulus intensity is critical in determining our perception. It is no accident that stimulus intensity is presented first in our quest to understand the relationship between the acoustic variables of sounds and how we perceive them.

In this section, we explore the many ways stimulus intensity influences a number of perceptual judgments we can make regarding the sounds we hear. We begin in Chapter 4 with defining the limits of our ability to detect the presence of a sound. We learn the minimum sound pressure levels that normal listeners need to judge a sound's presence. We learn how our ability to distinguish the presence of a sound from silence depends not only on its intensity, but on its frequency and how the sound is delivered to the listener. Chapter 5 explores the concept of loudness and answers a variety of questions. How is loudness defined? How do hearing scientists obtain loudness estimations from listeners?

How is loudness influenced by changes to a sound's intensity and frequency? Finally, we learn how hearing scientists attempt to explain why our loudness perceptions are the way they are.

This unit on intensity concludes with Chapter 6 on intensity discrimination. This chapter explores how sensitive we are to *changes* in stimulus intensity. In other words, what is the smallest difference in intensity between two sounds that normal listeners can just perceive? How do the intensity and frequency of a sound influence this ability? How do hearing scientists conduct experiments to measure this ability? How do hearing scientists explain our ability to detect very small changes in sound intensity?

4

AUDITORY SENSITIVITY

The important concepts you will learn in this chapter are:

- The relationships among auditory detection, absolute threshold, and auditory sensitivity.
- The measurement of absolute auditory thresholds in human listeners.
- The psychometric function.
- The relationship between audibility and sensitivity.
- Experimental findings regarding the limits of human auditory threshold.
- The effect of signal frequency on auditory sensitivity.
- The effect of listening conditions on auditory sensitivity.

Absolute Threshold

Audibility

Auditory Sensitivity

Comprehension

Detection

Discrimination

Minimum Audible Field (MAF)

Minimum Audible Pressure (MAP)

Monaural

Psychometric Function

Recognition

Sound Field

Threshold of Audibility

■ OVERVIEW

What determines our ability to "hear" a sound? Do the characteristics of some signals—their frequency, intensity, or duration—make them easier to hear than others? Most of us are familiar with dog whistles, which produce an auditory stimulus that most humans can't hear. Yet, if dogs are nearby, clearly they can hear it, as demonstrated by their response. Why can the dogs hear this particular stimulus, but we can't? Does how we listen to a sound matter? Could we hear better if we could listen with both ears, as opposed to just one? Does it matter if the sound comes through headphones as opposed to a loudspeaker? We explore the answers to these questions in this chapter.

■ DETECTION AND THE ABSOLUTE THRESHOLD

The most basic function of the auditory system is determining the presence of a sound. This, the lowest skill in the hierarchy of auditory behavior, we call **detection**. Before any further processing of the signal can occur, it must be audible to the listener. Detection is measured in terms of the **absolute threshold**, which is the magnitude of a stimulus necessary for the receiver to detect its presence 50 percent of the time. In other words, the listener must be able to correctly determine the presence of the signal half the time it is physically present. Absolute thresholds are not limited to the auditory system. Scientists interested in our other senses—sight, taste, and touch, for example—may also measure absolute thresholds for the detection of these stimuli in humans and other organisms.

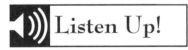 Listen Up!

HIERARCHY OF AUDITORY BEHAVIOR

Auditory perception is commonly described in terms of a hierarchy of behavior, which consists of four major levels of auditory ability.

1. **Detection** is the perception that something has occurred or that some state exists. In terms of auditory perception, detection implies the perception of the presence of a sound; it addresses the question, "Is the sound there?"

2. **Discrimination** is the process by which two stimuli, differing along some physical dimension, are responded to differentially. In the case of auditory perception, discrimination means that a listener judges as different either two different sounds presented to a listener or one sound that changes along some physical dimension. Before sounds can be discriminated, however, they must be detectable. Discrimination answers the question, "Did the sound change?"

3. **Recognition** is the awareness that something perceived has been perceived before. In terms of auditory perception, recognition implies that a sound is familiar and identifiable. It addresses the question, "What is this sound?" Before a sound can be recognized, it must first be audible, and we must be able to discriminate it from other sounds.

4. **Comprehension** answers the question, "What does this sound mean?" It is the process by which we extract meaning from sounds. For comprehension to occur, a sound must be detectable, we must be able to discriminate it from other sounds, and it must be familiar.

The four levels of auditory behavior (detection, discrimination, recognition, and comprehension) represent a serially ordered hierarchy. Each level builds on the preceding one.

MEASURING ABSOLUTE THRESHOLD AND THE PSYCHOMETRIC FUNCTION

As an example of how we might measure a detection threshold, suppose we are interested in knowing your absolute threshold for a sound. We present the sound repeatedly at a number of different intensities. Each time we present the sound, we keep a record of your response: "Did you hear it after the presentation? Did you not hear it after the presentation?"

Table 4-1 illustrates the results. In the table, we can see that you were able to detect the presence of the sound 50 percent of the time when it was delivered at an intensity of 15 dB SPL. This is your absolute threshold *for this particular sound.* Not all sounds you listen to will have an absolute threshold of 15 dB SPL; this is just an example. Also, when the sound was presented, you were required to say only whether it was present. You weren't required to describe it, and you didn't

TABLE 4-1 **Hypothetical Results from an Experiment to Measure Absolute Threshold.**

Intensity of the Sound (dB SPL)	Number of Times the Sound Was Heard	Total Number of Sound Presentations	Percentage of "Correct" Responses
5	0	10	0
10	3	10	30
15	5	10	50
20	7	10	70
25	10	10	100

have to decide whether it was the same or different from another sound; you only had to decide whether it was perceptible, compared to silence.

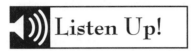 Listen Up!

PSYCHOMETRIC FUNCTIONS

A useful way of illustrating the results of the listening experiment shown in Table 4-1 is by means of a **psychometric function**. Psychometric functions plot some measure of our perception to a sound as a function of a physical parameter of the same sound. Figure 4-1 plots our hypothetical experimental results in terms of percentage-correct detection as a function of sound intensity. Look at the intersecting dashed lines in that figure and where they cross the psychometric function.

- On the *y*-axis, the line crosses the 50 percent performance point, the typical performance criterion for absolute threshold.

- On the *x*-axis, the line intersects the function at a sound pressure level equivalent to 15 dB SPL, which represents your absolute threshold for this sound.

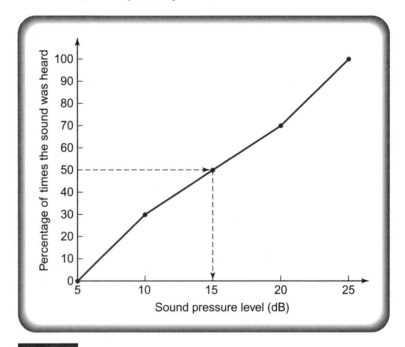

FIGURE 4-1 Psychometric Function Summarizing the Results of a
Listening Experiment Performance of Detection: The
percentage of correct responses is plotted as a function
of stimulus intensity.

The psychometric function is very useful in illustrating how our perceptions to sounds change as we change a physical parameter of a stimulus. We use the concept of the psychometric function in later chapters as we explore higher levels of auditory processing.

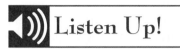 Listen Up!

PERFORMANCE CRITERIA FOR AUDITORY THRESHOLDS

All auditory thresholds are determined relative to a preselected percentage-correct performance level. Whether they are thresholds of detection, discrimination, recognition, or comprehension, some performance-level criterion, in terms of percentage correct, is used. The actual level of performance, however, may vary depending on the level of auditory behavior required of the listener. In the case of detection, performance is usually determined at 50 percent. As we will see, thresholds of higher levels of auditory behavior are determined using other levels of performance that are usually higher than 50 percent.

AUDIBILITY AND SENSITIVITY

The terms **audibility** and **auditory sensitivity** are used by hearing scientists to describe the limits of our hearing detection capability. Audibility and sensitivity relate to an absolute threshold, that is, under ideal circumstances, the lowest sound pressure level required to detect the presence of a given sound.

- Given a particular sound, a *low absolute threshold*, measured in dB, suggests that we require less stimulus intensity to perceive it. These sounds are described as having a high degree of audibility; they are *easy* to hear.

- A *high absolute threshold* for a sound means that we require relatively greater sound intensities to detect its presence. These sounds are described as having a low degree of audibility; they are *hard* to hear.

Sensitivity and audibility are *inversely* related to the magnitude of absolute threshold. In other words:

- If audibility is poor (a high threshold), our sensitivity is considered poor as well.

- If audibility is good (a low threshold), our sensitivity is described as good.

Low threshold is equivalent to having good sensitivity and audibility. High threshold is equivalent to having poor sensitivity and audibility.

■ PREVIOUS STUDIES OF NORMAL HUMAN AUDITORY SENSITIVITY

The lower limits of human auditory sensitivity were investigated nearly a century ago. Perhaps the most cited report of human sensitivity comes from Sivian and White (1933). In this classic study, the researchers had normal-hearing subjects, mostly young adults, listen to a variety of pure tones under several different listening conditions. They presented many pure tones at different frequencies and measured the intensities of the pure tones at the points where the subjects could just detect their presence. The absolute thresholds of detection were analyzed as a function of the frequency of the pure tones.

How the sounds were delivered to the listeners was another important variable in their study. When this report was published, two listening conditions, or modes of listening, were of interest to hearing scientists:

1. One listening mode was *binaurally* in a **sound field**. In this condition, the subjects were seated in a special sound chamber, 1 m away from a loudspeaker, which was the sound source for the pure tones. Both ears of the listener were allowed to participate in the test; that is, neither ear was blocked or occluded in any way. Sivian and White contend that this is the way we typically encounter sounds in the real world.

2. The second listening mode was *monaurally under headphones*. With this sound presentation, the pure tones were delivered to one side of the headphones that were worn by the subjects and that were similar to the headphones audiologists currently use in clinical testing. Because the sounds were presented to one side only, only one ear participated in the test; hence this listening condition was **monaural**.

In reporting the results of their study, Sivian and White combined their findings with older studies related to auditory sensitivity measured in similar listening conditions. Figure 4-2 is based on their published report. In that figure absolute thresholds, in dB SPL, are plotted as a function of the frequency of the delivered pure tones. It is a compilation of the results from Sivian and White and other experimental data gathered before 1933. Notice that the range of frequencies represented is quite large: 60 Hz through 15,000 Hz. This is why the frequency axis is represented on a logarithmic scale. The two curves represent the two modes of listening, which are the parameters of the graph. The curve marked MAP (**minimum audible pressure**) refers to the monaural headphone presentation. The curve marked MAF (**minimum audible field**) refers to the binaural sound field presentation. These thresholds have become known as **threshold of audibility** curves. These functions, or curves, represent the lowest limits of normal human auditory sensitivity.

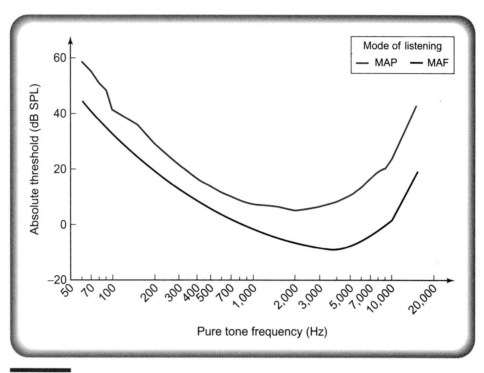

FIGURE 4-2 Absolute Thresholds as a Function of Pure Tone Frequency and Listening Condition. (From Sivian and White, 1933.)

WHAT THE SIVIAN AND WHITE RESULTS TELL US ABOUT NORMAL HUMAN AUDITORY SENSITIVITY

Sivian and White's report, as well as others that followed, are important because they illustrate that human auditory sensitivity depends not only on the characteristics of the sounds we listen to but also how we listen to them. The significance of their findings fall into two categories:

1. The Effect of Frequency on Absolute Thresholds.
2. The Effect of Mode of Listening on Absolute Thresholds.

The Effect of Frequency on Absolute Thresholds

In Figure 4-2, both curves demonstrate the same effect of frequency on the auditory thresholds. The absolute thresholds for the lowest pure tone frequencies are relatively high (high thresholds correspond to poor sensitivity and reduced audibility). As the frequency of the pure tones increases, auditory thresholds decrease (our sensitivity to higher-frequency pure tones increases and the audibility of these tones improves). Note the frequency range in which the absolute thresholds are at their lowest values:

generally 1,000 Hz through 5,000 Hz. This suggests that our best sensitivity occurs within this range. As the frequency of the pure tones increases above 5,000 Hz, auditory thresholds increase, and, as the frequency of the pure tones decreases below 1,000 Hz, auditory thresholds increase. This suggests that our sensitivity to these signals decreases and that the audibility of these tones becomes poorer. The important conclusion is that human auditory sensitivity is *not constant* across frequency. We are most sensitive to sounds characterized by energy between 1,000 Hz and 5,000 Hz. The farther away the signal's frequency is from our most sensitive region—either higher or lower in frequency—the poorer our sensitivity becomes.

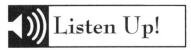 Listen Up!

AUDIBILITY BEYOND THE BOUNDARIES OF SIVIAN AND WHITE

Sivian and White illustrate normal thresholds of audibility between the frequencies 60 Hz and 15,000 Hz. Subsequent studies (Corso, 1963; von Bekesy, 1960) demonstrate our audibility for sounds below 60 Hz and above 10,000 Hz. A compilation of the results of these studies is provided in Figure 4-3. In that figure, absolute thresholds are plotted as a function

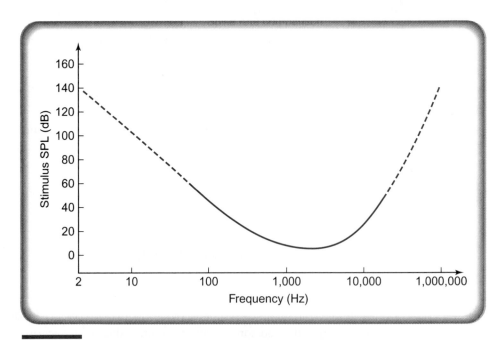

FIGURE 4-3 Absolute Thresholds as a Function of Pure Tone Frequency in the MAP Condition: This figure includes data from several experiments interested in normal human sensitivity to pure tones throughout a very broad frequency range. (From Small, 1973.)

of pure tone signal frequency. The solid part of the function denotes the MAP thresholds reported by Sivian and White. The dashed part illustrates normal human absolute thresholds in the MAP listening mode compiled from von Bekesy and Corso. Notice that the main conclusion from Sivian and White regarding our change in sensitivity with change in frequency holds for pure tone frequencies below 60 Hz and above 15,000 Hz. In other words, the farther away signal frequency is from our most sensitive frequency region, the poorer our sensitivity becomes.

The Effect of Mode of Listening on Absolute Thresholds

Recall that the two functions illustrated in Figure 4-2 represent the two ways the subjects received their signals: monaural headphone delivery (MAP) and binaural sound field delivery (MAF). The figure clearly shows that the MAF listening mode demonstrates the lower absolute thresholds, compared to the MAP listening mode—for the entire range of signal frequencies presented to the listeners. This finding suggests that our sensitivity to sound is always better when we listen with both ears in a sound field condition, regardless of the frequency of the sound. Listening with just one ear, through headphones, results in reduced sensitivity. The sounds are not as audible.

Why is this? Hearing scientists agree that most of the differences in thresholds between the MAP and MAF curves are due to the fact that, in the MAF condition, subjects are listening binaurally and that, in the MAP condition, subjects are listening monaurally. Apparently, our ability to detect the presence of a sound improves considerably if we are allowed to listen with both ears, as opposed to just one. As we explore more complex perceptions to sounds, we will see that this is almost always the case. Two ears are better than one, regardless of the listening task.

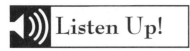

THE HEARING LEVEL REFERENCE AND THE MAP CURVE

Recall from Chapter 3 that the hearing level (HL) decibel scale is based on average, normal-hearing sensitivity, which is taken as the MAP threshold of audibility curve reported by Sivian and White. Why is the MAP curve used rather than the MAF audibility curve? In clinical settings, a listener's detection ability is usually measured monaurally under headphones, not binaurally in sound field. Hence, the MAP curve better illustrates the typical listening mode in clinical testing, and so using this reference for threshold of audibility makes sense.

When an individual requests a hearing test from an audiologist, the primary focus is on how the person's hearing compares to that of normal-hearing listeners. The question is not how the individual's hearing changes as a function of frequency. The MAP threshold of audibility curve provides audiologists with a reference for normal hearing, which accounts for the normal variation in threshold we expect as the frequency of the sound changes. In fact, when thresholds from normal-hearing listeners are plotted in dB HL, the function is a straight line at 0 dB across frequency.

Although monaural versus binaural listening accounts for much of the difference in absolute thresholds between the MAP and MAF threshold of audibility curves, it doesn't account for all of it. In Figure 4-2, when signal frequencies fall between 1,000 Hz and 5,000 Hz, the MAP and MAF curves diverge. In other words, the difference in absolute thresholds between these two listening conditions becomes greater. Some characteristic of these sounds improves their audibility between these two listening modes. Scientists suggest that the reason has to do with the fact that, in the MAF listening mode, the signal is allowed to physically interact with the body, head, pinna, and open ear canal of the listener. This is not the case in the MAP condition, in which the signal originates at the entrance of the ear canal, and in which, more importantly, the ear canal is closed, or occluded, by the headphone. When some sound waves are allowed to physically interact with the body, head, pinna, and ear canal of the listener, they generate a higher sound pressure level by the time they reach the eardrum, compared to their sound pressure level at the source.

The sounds that benefit most by this boost in amplitude are determined by their frequency. It just so happens that sounds with frequencies between 1,000 Hz and 5,000 Hz are the most affected by the physical interaction that occurs with the human body seated some distance away from the sound source. In other words, the intensity of these sounds, as they reach the end of the outer ear canal, is increased, compared to their intensity at the source. Remember that, when sound intensity is increased (even slightly), sensitivity and audibility improve. When the sound is delivered directly to the entrance of the ear canal, as in the MAP listening mode, it can't physically interact with the body, head, and pinna.

The studies of human sensitivity discussed in this chapter indicate the following important conclusions:

1. Our ability to detect a signal depends primarily on its frequency and intensity. Human listeners are most sensitive to sounds within the 1,000-Hz through 5,000-Hz frequency region. We are better able to detect the presence of these sounds at lower intensity levels compared to sounds that fall outside this frequency region. In other words, depending on their

frequency, some sounds at a given intensity level may be audible, but other sounds may not. In the case of the dog whistle, dogs have thresholds of detection that are significantly different from those of human listeners. They are especially more sensitive to the presence of high-frequency sounds than we are.

2. Our sensitivity to sounds also depends on how they are presented. If we are allowed to listen with both ears, as opposed to just one ear, sensitivity and audibility improve. If the sound wave is delivered in such a way as to allow physical interaction with the human body, head, pinna, and open ear canal, sensitivity and audibility improve, compared to delivery systems that restrict the physical interaction between the sound wave and the listener. Detection represents the most basic skill of the human auditory system, but the stimulus and listening variables affecting this skill are complex.

■ CHAPTER SUMMARY

We have covered several important concepts related to normal human auditory sensitivity. After reading and studying this chapter, you should be able to do the following:

- Provide definitions of auditory detection, absolute threshold, auditory sensitivity, and audibility.

- Describe how detection, absolute threshold, sensitivity, and audibility are related.

- Describe how absolute auditory thresholds are measured in humans and represented in terms of a psychometric function.

- Describe the experimental conditions and results reported by Sivian and White.

- Define minimal audible pressure and minimal audible field.

- Explain the concept of the threshold of audibility curve.

- Describe the effect of signal frequency on normal human auditory sensitivity.

- Describe the effect of listening conditions on normal human auditory sensitivity.

- Explain how monaural versus binaural listening impacts normal human auditory sensitivity.

- Explain how earphone versus sound field delivery of signals impacts normal human auditory sensitivity.

REFERENCES

Corso, J. F. "Bone Conducted Thresholds for Sonic and Ultrasonic Frequencies." *Journal of the Acoustical Society of America* 35 (1963): 1738–1743.

Sivian, L. J., and S. D. White. "On Minimum Audible Sound Fields." *Journal of the Acoustical Society of America* 4 (1933): 288–321.

Small, A. M. "Psychoacoustics." In *Normal Aspects of Speech, Hearing, and Language*, 1st ed., edited by F. D. Minifie, T. J. Hixon, and F. Williams, 343–420. Upper Saddle River, NJ: Prentice Hall, 1973.

von Bekesy, G. *Experiments in Hearing.* New York: McGraw-Hill, 1960.

5

LOUDNESS

LEARNING OBJECTIVES

The important concepts you will learn
in this chapter are:

- The definition of loudness.
- The difference between auditory
  perception and stimulus variables.
- The effect of stimulus intensity on
  loudness perception.
- The experimental procedures used
  by hearing scientists to obtain
  estimates of loudness from human
  listeners.
- The two units of loudness
  estimation.
- Equal loudness contours.
- The effect of stimulus frequency
  on loudness.
- Differences in loudness growth for
  low- and high-frequency tones.
- The use of excitation patterns
  as a model to explain loudness
  perception.

KEY TERMS

Direct Magnitude
  Estimation (DME)
Direct Magnitude
  Production (DMP)
Equal Loudness Contour
Excitation Pattern
Experimental Paradigm
Indirect Method of
  Loudness Estimation

Loudness
Loudness Balance
  Procedure
Model
Ordinal Scale
Phons
Ratio Scale
Sone
Wideband Noise

OVERVIEW

Loudness is the perceptual quality of sound related to intensity. All of us understand that sounds can be judged as faint, comfortably loud, or uncomfortably loud. When we use these terms to describe a sound, we are describing our perception of its magnitude, or strength. What stimulus parameters determine our perception of loudness? We all would predict that, as we increase the physical intensity of a sound, our perception of its loudness increases. But what if we hold the sound's intensity constant and change its frequency? Does loudness stay the same or change? If we increase the intensity of a low-frequency tone, is the growth in loudness the same as for a high-frequency tone? We explore these issues in this chapter.

PERCEPTION VERSUS STIMULUS VARIABLES

Hearing scientists must understand the difference between measuring our perceptions of a sound and measuring a physical parameter of a sound. The two types of measurement are not the same. Loudness is a psychological perception that we attribute to sound, not something that can be measured directly. In other words, scientists can't directly measure your perception of loudness by attaching a measuring device to your ear as you listen to a sound. Rather, they must rely on your interpretation or description—your estimation—of a sound. So, to measure loudness, scientists must have a listener.

This is not the case with the measurement of the physical acoustic variables of sound, such as intensity, frequency, duration, and phase. Scientists can measure these parameters of sound in the absence of a human listener. This fact has a number of implications regarding the measurement of loudness perception, both in how we collect loudness estimates from listeners and in the units of loudness that we derive from such experimental procedures.

STIMULUS INTENSITY AND ITS EFFECT ON LOUDNESS

We don't need to take a course in psychoacoustics to realize that as we increase the intensity of a sound, our estimation of its loudness grows. However, as we examine the experimental evidence related to this relationship, we learn how scientists measure loudness perception in human listeners and the relationship between stimulus intensity and loudness. Two basic methods are the direct magnitude estimation and direct production estimation procedures.

DIRECT MAGNITUDE ESTIMATION

A study by Stevens and Tulving (1957) illustrates the effect of stimulus intensity on loudness and provides an example of one way in which scientists obtain loudness estimates from human listeners. In this study, 70 untrained young adults listened to pairs of noise stimuli. The type of noise they heard was **wideband noise,** which is a complex stimulus characterized by a continuous spectrum that is flat throughout the audible frequency range. The first wideband noise stimulus was presented at 85 dB SPL. The second was presented at 55, 65, 75, 85, 90, 95, 100, or 105 dB SPL. The subjects' task was to listen to the first noise at 85 dB SPL, and then listen to the second noise and assign a number to the loudness of the *second* noise. The listeners were told that the loudness of the first noise was equivalent to 10. So if they thought that the second noise was twice as loud as the first, they should assign a value of 20. Likewise, if the listeners judged the second noise to be half as loud as the first sound, they should assign a value of 5.

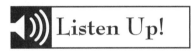 Listen Up!

USING EXPERIMENTAL PARADIGM FIGURES

In the many experiments related to human auditory perception, the listening conditions that subjects are presented with are easily represented in terms of the experimental paradigm. The **experimental paradigm** is a schematic representation of the number, duration, frequency, or intensity of the sounds presented to the subjects as a function of time. The judgments that the listener supplies regarding the stimuli may also be included in the schematic.

Figure 5-1 illustrates the experimental paradigm used by Stevens and Tulving. Two stimuli—the standard stimulus and the variable stimulus—are presented to the listener along the abscissa, which represents time. The intensities of the stimuli are represented on the ordinate. The reference stimulus has a loudness of 10, as set by the experimenters. The variable stimulus is randomly set to one of eight intensities, ranging from 55 through

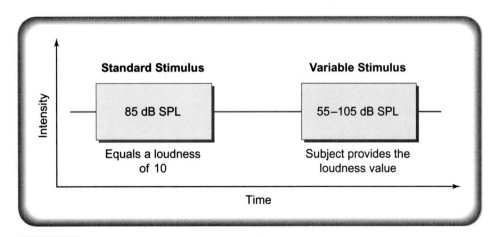

FIGURE 5-1 **Experimental Paradigm of a Direct Magnitude Estimation (DME) Loudness Procedure: This is the experimental design used by Stevens and Tulving (1957) to address the effect of wideband noise intensity on loudness perception. See text for further information concerning this procedure.**

105 dB SPL. With each presentation of the noise pairs, the subjects were required to assign a number corresponding to the loudness of the variable, based on their perceived loudness.

The experimental results from Stevens and Tulving are illustrated in Figure 5-2. The average judgments of loudness magnitude, as provided by the 70 listeners, are plotted as a function of the intensity, dB SPL, of the variable stimulus, which was the second wideband noise presented in the stimulus pair. The intensity of the standard stimulus is marked on the figure as *standard*. It is clear that, as the intensity of the variable stimulus increases from 55 through 105 dB SPL, the magnitude of the loudness estimate increases. More importantly, the growth of loudness estimation is linearly related to the increase in stimulus intensity. Just look at the function (a straight-line) relating the two experimental variables. We conclude from these results that not only does our loudness perception increase with increases in stimulus intensity, but also that the growth of loudness is *linear*, or proportional, to the increase in intensity. In other words, with each unit increase in stimulus intensity, the magnitude of the loudness estimate increases by a proportional amount.

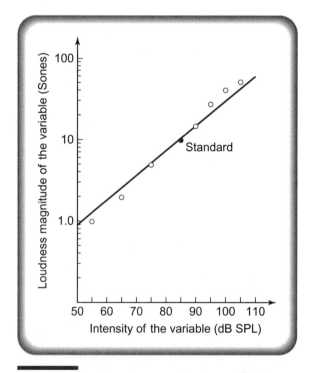

FIGURE 5-2 Judgments of Loudness Magnitude as a
Function of Wideband Noise Intensity.
(From Stevens and Tulving, 1933.)

Stevens and Tulving's experimental paradigm (Figure 5-1) is an example of a **direct magnitude estimation (DME)** procedure. The subjects participating in this study were required to provide a ratio estimate of the loudness of the second noise based on their comparisons to the loudness of the first noise. Listeners were instructed to judge the loudness of the second sound based on the loudness of the first sound, which equaled 10. The numbers on the ordinate of Figure 5-2, loudness magnitude estimate, represent a **ratio scale**, which is a scale in which two variables of interest, in this case stimulus intensity and loudness, are *proportional*. A ratio scale also implies that mathematical operations, such as multiplication and division, are meaningful and that there is a *true* zero. (This is not the case with other procedures used to estimate loudness.) When a direct procedure is used to estimate loudness:

- A sound with a loudness estimate of 10 is twice as loud as a sound with a loudness estimate of 5.

- A sound with a loudness estimate of 10 is only half as loud as a sound with a loudness estimate of 20.

- Zero (0) means the absence of loudness.

Direct magnitude estimation procedures of loudness are therefore very powerful because they provide a ratio scale relating loudness estimation and stimulus intensity.

DIRECT MAGNITUDE PRODUCTION

Another experimental procedure for directly estimating loudness that also yields a ratio scale is **direct magnitude production (DMP)**. An example of a DMP experimental paradigm is shown in Figure 5-3. In DMP, subjects listen to pairs of stimuli. The first stimulus, the standard, is presented at a fixed intensity.

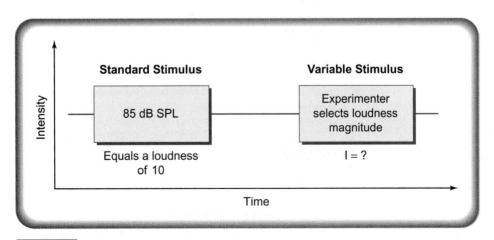

FIGURE 5-3 Experimental Paradigm of a Direct Magnitude Production (DMP) Loudness Procedure.

The listener is told to equate the loudness of this sound to an arbitrary value, such as 10.

The DMP procedure differs from DME, however, in that the *listener* controls the intensity of the second stimulus. The experimenter asks the listener to adjust the intensity of the second sound to a preselected loudness estimate value and then collects data on the intensity of the second stimulus that the listener chooses. For example, the first stimulus is presented at 85 dB SPL, and the listener is told to equate the loudness of this sound to 10. The experimenter then presents the second stimulus to the listener with the instructions to adjust the intensity of this sound to a loudness of 20, which the listener judges to be twice as loud as the first. The intensity of the second variable sound is then paired with the loudness estimation magnitude of 20. The experiment continues, with the experimenter requiring subjects to pair other loudness values with the stimulus intensities provided by the listener so as to match the required loudness estimation. Both direct magnitude estimation and direct magnitude production procedures of loudness yield a ratio scale relating loudness estimation and stimulus intensity.

UNITS OF LOUDNESS ESTIMATION

How do hearing scientists represent the loudness estimates that they obtain from human listeners? In what units do they measure the estimates? For loudness estimates obtained using a direct procedure of loudness estimation (DME or DMP), the unit assigned is the sone. One **sone** is equivalent to the loudness of a 1,000-Hz tone presented 40 dB above the listener's threshold at 1,000 Hz. Because the sone is tied to direct procedures of loudness estimation, a sound with a loudness of 10 sones is, by definition, half as loud as a sound with a loudness equivalent to 20 sones. Likewise, a sound with a loudness of 1 sone is one-fifth as loud as a sound with a loudness of 5 sones.

The unit used for stimulus intensity, the decibel (dB), is *never* used as a unit of loudness estimation. Stimulus variables are physical quantities that can be measured independently of a human observer. On the other hand, psychological perceptions, like loudness, are obtained from judgments of a human observer based on some perceptual characteristic of the sound.

■ STIMULUS FREQUENCY AND ITS EFFECT ON LOUDNESS

So the intensity of a stimulus is a very important variable in determining our perception of loudness, but is it the only one? For example, if we keep the intensity of a sound constant and change its frequency from very low to very high, does loudness change? If it does, how does it change? To help answer these questions, we visit one of the earliest studies investigating loudness perceptions of pure tones at a variety of frequencies and intensities.

Fletcher and Munson (1933), scientists working at Bell Telephone Laboratories nearly a century ago, published a report in 1933 of several studies they conducted concerning the loudness of simple and complex sounds. In one portion of their report, they describe an experiment in which 11 normal-hearing listeners were presented with 10 different pure tones, ranging in frequency from 62 Hz to 16,000 Hz and in intensity from nearly audible to more than 100 dB above threshold. The subjects listened to the pure tones paired with a 1,000-Hz reference tone. The 1,000-Hz reference tone, under the experimenters' control, ranged in intensity from 10 dB SL (sensation level) to 110 dB SL. With each stimulus pair, the subjects were required to judge which of the tones was louder: the reference tone or the variable tone. From their observations, Fletcher and Munson were able to calculate the intensity of the variable tone having *equal loudness* to the reference tone.

This type of loudness estimation has become known as the **loudness balance procedure**. Figure 5-4 shows an example. The experimental paradigm for a traditional loudness balance procedure presents a listener with two stimuli in succession. The experimenter sets the properties of the first stimulus, the reference. In Figure 5-4, the reference stimulus is a 1,000-Hz pure tone at an intensity equivalent to 20 dB SL. The experimenter also determines the frequency of the second stimulus, the variable. In Figure 5-4, the frequency of the variable is 250 Hz. The listener's task is to adjust the intensity of the variable stimulus so that it is *as loud as* the reference. The subject may either physically control the intensity of the variable stimulus or simply tell the experimenter to make the variable stimulus intensity higher or lower. How the subject controls the variable intensity isn't important. What is important is that the variable intensity, in the end, is equal to the loudness of the reference. The experimenter records the frequency and intensity of the

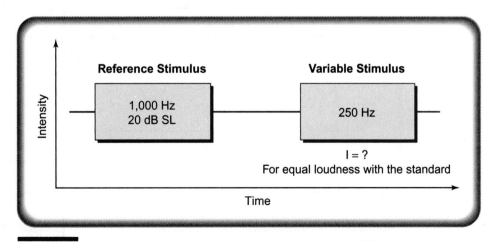

FIGURE 5-4 Experimental Paradigm of a Loudness Balance Procedure When the Reference Stimulus Is at 20 dB SL.

variable stimulus necessary for equal loudness to a 1,000-Hz reference tone, which remains fixed at a predetermined intensity.

During the loudness balance procedure, the subject must ignore pitch differences between the standard and variable stimuli, because these sounds usually have different frequencies. The subjects are to pay attention only to the loudness of the two tones and make them equal. They must focus on adjusting the loudness of the reference tone to make it equal to that of the variable tone.

GENERATING AN EQUAL LOUDNESS CONTOUR USING A LOUDNESS BALANCE PROCEDURE

Look at the experimental procedure illustrated in Figure 5-5. A typical loudness balance procedure is performed with a normal-hearing listener.

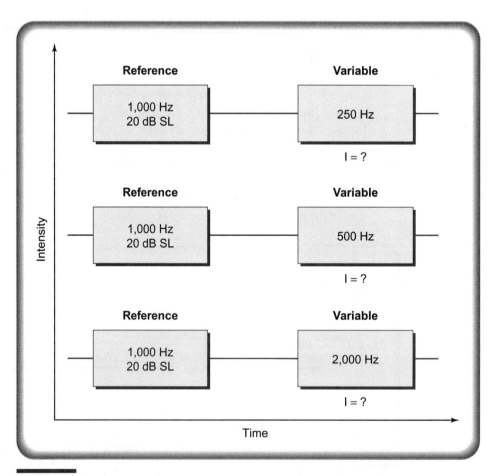

FIGURE 5-5 Experimental Paradigm of a Loudness Balance Procedure When the Reference Stimulus Is at 20 dB SL and the Frequency of the Variable Stimulus Changes Throughout the Course of the Experiment.

- The reference tone is a 1,000-Hz pure tone 20 dB above the listener's absolute threshold at 1,000 Hz, or 20 dB SL. In the top panel, the reference stimulus is paired with a variable tone at 250 Hz. The subject adjusts the intensity of the 250-Hz variable tone so that it is equal to the loudness of the reference. The experimenter records the intensity of the variable tone judged by the listener as equally loud as the reference. (This is identical to the stimulus paradigm shown in Figure 5-4.)

- Next the experimenter changes the frequency of the variable tone to 500 Hz, as illustrated in the middle panel of Figure 5-5. This new variable tone is paired with the reference tone, still 1,000 Hz at 20 dB SL. Again, the subject is required to provide an intensity of the 500-Hz variable tone that results in equal loudness to the reference. The experimenter records the intensity of the variable tone provided by the subject.

- The experimenter changes the frequency of the variable stimulus again, as represented in the bottom panel of the figure. This time, the variable tone is presented at a frequency of 2,000 Hz. The balance procedure is repeated a third time.

The experimenter repeats this procedure again and again, selecting variable pure tone frequencies ranging from 20 Hz to 16,000 Hz. Each variable tone is paired with the 1,000-Hz reference tone at 20 dB SL. The results of this loudness balance procedure are illustrated in Figure 5-6 and come from Fletcher and Munson's 1933

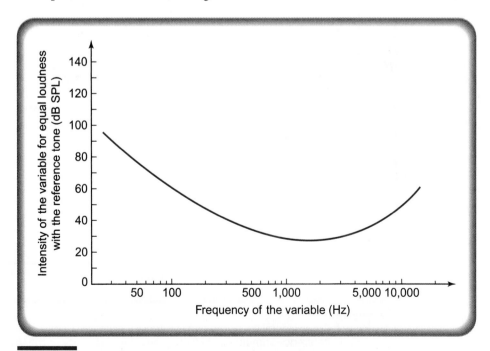

FIGURE 5-6 Equal Loudness Contour for a 20-dB SL Reference. (After Fletcher and Munson, 1933.)

report. This figure plots the intensity of the variable tone necessary for equal loudness to the reference tone as a function of the variable tone's frequency. The resulting function is called an **equal loudness contour**. Every stimulus falling on this function has, by definition, equal loudness to the 1,000-Hz, 20-dB-SL reference tone. Therefore, every variable stimulus falling on this function has equal loudness with every other and a loudness equivalent to a 1,000-Hz pure tone slightly above detection threshold.

Suppose the experimenter wants to make another equal loudness contour using a different reference tone? The experimental paradigm for the new contour is illustrated in Figure 5-7. In this case, loudness estimates are obtained using a 1,000-Hz reference tone 60 dB above absolute threshold. The higher-intensity

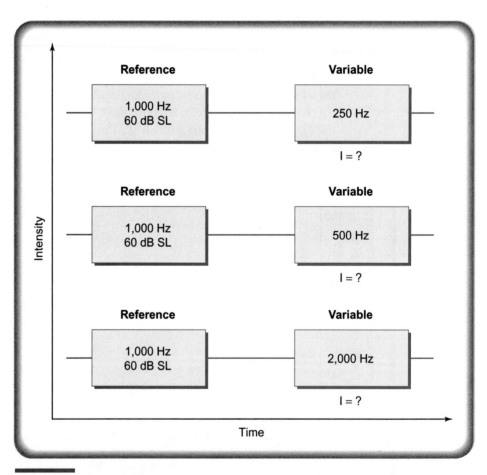

FIGURE 5-7 **Experimental Paradigm of a Loudness Balance Procedure When the Reference Stimulus is at 60 dB SL and the Frequency of the Variable Stimulus Changes Throughout the Course of the Experiment.**

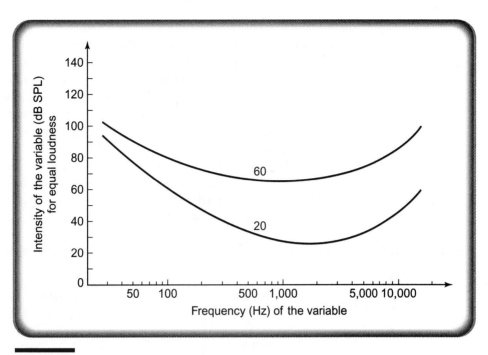

FIGURE 5-8 Equal Loudness Contours for a 20- and 60-dB SL Reference. (After Fletcher and Munson, 1933.)

reference tone is paired with three variable tone frequencies, as illustrated in the three panels of the figure. For each variable tone frequency, the listener adjusts the intensity of the variable to match the loudness of the reference, and the experimenter records the intensity that the listener requires to make the variable equal to the loudness of the reference tone.

The results from the second loudness balance procedure are added to the first procedure and represented in Figure 5-8. In this figure, the intensity of the variable tone necessary for equal loudness to the reference is plotted as a function of the variable tone frequency. Again, these results come from Fletcher and Munson. The figure shows two separate functions, or equal loudness contours. The bottom function (20) represents data reflecting equal loudness to a 20-dB-SL, 1,000-Hz reference. The other (60) represents data reflecting equal loudness to a 60-dB-SL, 1,000-Hz reference tone.

How can we compare these two equal loudness contours? The variable stimuli falling on the 60 contour are *louder* than the variable stimuli associated with the 20 contour. This makes sense because the intensity of the reference tone used to generate the 60 contour is higher than the reference tone used to generate the 20 contour. As the study by Stevens and Tulving showed, as we increase stimulus intensity, loudness increases as well. However, we can't say that the variable tones falling on the 60 equal loudness contour are *three times as loud* as the variable tones falling on the 20 contour. Loudness estimates obtained from a loudness balance procedure don't provide a ratio relationship between loudness and the reference stimulus intensity. Rather, they provide an **ordinal scale**, in which the magnitude of the loudness estimates can be ordered from low to high, but without a ratio relationship. In an ordinal scale, comparisons can be made of greater and lesser and of equality and inequality. Mathematical operations of addition and subtraction, however, are meaningless.

To complete our loudness balance experiment, the experimenter wants to generate one more equal loudness contour, this time with a high-intensity standard stimulus. Figure 5-9 illustrates the experimental paradigm used to generate this third equal loudness contour. The experimenter pairs three variable frequencies with a

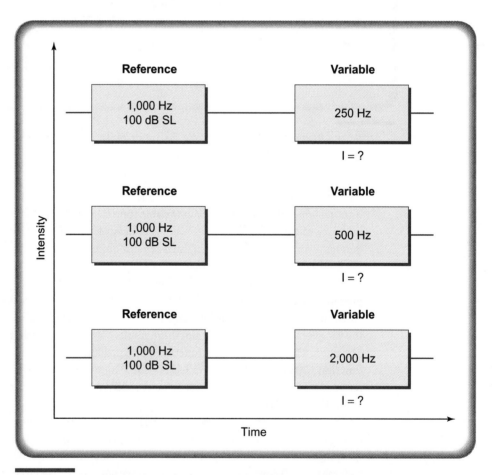

FIGURE 5-9 Experimental Paradigm of a Loudness Balance Procedure When the Reference Stimulus is at 100 dB SL and the Frequency of the Variable Stimulus Changes Throughout the Course of the Experiment.

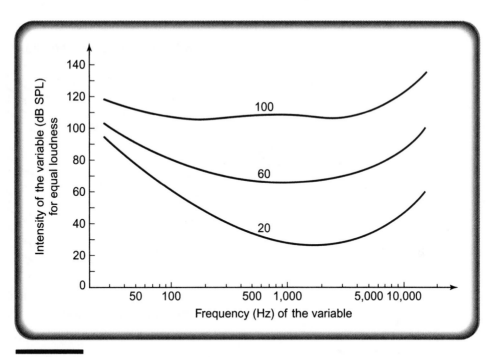

FIGURE 5-10 Equal Loudness Contours for a 20-, 60-, and 100-dB SL Reference. (After Fletcher and Munson, 1933.)

1,000-Hz reference 100 dB above the subject's absolute threshold at 1,000 Hz. For each variable pure tone frequency, the listener adjusts the intensity of the variable tone to match the loudness of the 100-dB-SL reference, and the experimenter records the intensity and frequency of the variable tone, as provided by the subject, that results in equal loudness to the reference tone.

Figure 5-10 adds the results of this last loudness balance procedure to the cumulative plot, which is again derived from the results reported by Fletcher and Munson for a range of variable pure tone frequencies. As before, the intensity of each variable tone, as judged by the listener to have equal loudness with the 1,000-Hz, 100-dB-SL reference, is plotted as a function of the variable tone frequency. The figure now shows three separate equal loudness contours.

1. One (20) represents equal loudness to a 1,000-Hz, 20-dB-SL reference.

2. A second (60) represents equal loudness to a 1,000-Hz, 60-dB-SL reference tone.

3. The last (100) represents equal loudness to a 1,000-Hz, 100-dB-SL reference.

As before, we can rank-order these contours in terms of their loudness. The variable tones falling on the 100 contour are louder than those falling on the 60 and 20 contours, but we can't say *how much louder*.

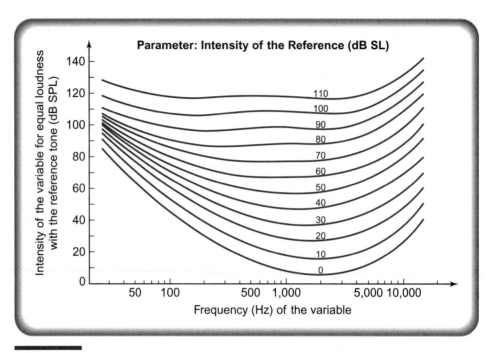

FIGURE 5-11 Loudness Level as a Function of Variable Frequency and Reference Intensity: Each curve is an equal loudness contour. (From Fletcher and Munson, 1933.)

FLETCHER AND MUNSON'S EQUAL LOUDNESS CONTOURS

Recall that Fletcher and Munson investigated equal loudness contours using 1,000-Hz reference tones ranging in intensity from 10 dB SL to 110 dB SPL. An idealized representation of their results is provided in Figure 5-11. This figure represents 12 separate equal loudness contours, numbered 0–110. This is the parameter of the graph. The numbers reflecting the parameter indicate the intensity (dB SL) of the 1,000-Hz reference tone, that is, the intensity of the reference tone that is 10–110 dB above the listeners' absolute threshold at 1,000 Hz. Each contour plots the intensity of the variable pure tone necessary for equal loudness with the reference stimulus as a function of the variable tone frequency. The 0 contour represents thresholds of audibility as a function of frequency. This contour, derived from Sivian and White's (1933) MAP data, is provided for comparison regarding the loudness perceptions of tones presented to listeners above thresholds of detection.

UNITS OF LOUDNESS ESTIMATION USING A LOUDNESS BALANCE PROCEDURE

The loudness balance procedure is an example of an **indirect method of loudness estimation**, which contrasts with direct procedures of loudness estimation, such as DME and DMP. Whereas direct methods of loudness estimation provide loudness units that reflect ratio scaling, indirect methods involve loudness units that reflect ordinal scaling.

This important difference determines how the loudness estimates derived from either procedure may be compared. Sones, the units of loudness obtained from a direct procedure, may be added, subtracted, multiplied, and divided with meaning because they are established by the listener, providing a ratio relationship between stimulus intensity and its loudness. This is not the case with loudness estimates obtained from indirect procedures, such as loudness balance. In these procedures, listeners are relating the loudness of a tone with a reference only *when they are the same*. They do not provide intensities of the variable tone judged as twice as loud, half as loud, or in any other comparison to the reference sound. As a result, using indirect procedures of loudness estimation, we can establish a relationship between loudness and intensity only at one point: when the loudness of the tones is equal.

Therefore, the loudness units for direct and indirect procedures of loudness estimation are different. Loudness estimates obtained from indirect procedures are expressed in the units of **phons**, which, unlike sones, can't be added, subtracted, multiplied, or divided. They can only be *ranked*.

Look again at Fletcher and Munson's equal loudness contours in Figure 5-11. Recall that the parameter in this figure refers to the intensity of the reference tone, as well as to the magnitude of the loudness estimate, in phons. For example, the variable tones falling on the 40 contour have a loudness equivalent to 40 phons, and the variable tones falling on the 80 contour have a loudness equivalent to 80 phons. Eighty phons is louder than 40 phons, but 80 phons is not necessarily twice as loud as 40 phons.

WHAT FLETCHER AND MUNSON TELL US ABOUT THE EFFECT OF FREQUENCY ON LOUDNESS

To determine the effect of frequency on loudness perception, one approach is to compare the *shape* of Fletcher and Munson's equal loudness contours when the intensity of the reference stimulus is low, medium, and high. Figure 5-10 shows the equal loudness contours corresponding to 20, 60, and 100 phons. These contours represent conditions in which the reference intensity is low (20 phons), medium (60 phons), and high (100 phons). Clearly the shapes of these three contours aren't parallel. As the loudness of the reference stimulus increases, the contours flatten. In other words, for sounds characterized as, say, "soft," as the frequency of the sound increases from very low frequencies to higher frequencies, the intensity of the variable tone decreases in order to maintain soft loudness. As the frequency of the soft sound increases above about 2,000 Hz, the intensity must be increased to maintain loudness. On the other hand, very loud sounds demonstrate little variation in intensity as variable frequency changes from 20 Hz through 16,000 Hz in order to maintain loudness.

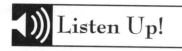

A PRACTICAL EXERCISE TO EXPLORE LOUDNESS CHANGE WITH FREQUENCY FOR LOW-, MEDIUM-, AND HIGH-INTENSITY SOUNDS

Place a clear ruler *horizontally* across Figure 5-11, connecting the ordinate axis markers corresponding to a variable intensity of 30 dB SPL. Now move your finger along the ruler's straight edge across the abscissa (the variable frequency) from the lefthand end of the axis (20 Hz) through the righthand end of the axis (16,000 Hz). *Pay attention to the loudness contours you cross as you sweep your finger through the variable frequencies.*

This exercise gives you an idea of your loudness perceptions of the sounds as you keep the intensity constant while steadily increasing the frequency.

- You should discover that the 30-dB-SPL tone is below absolute threshold until the variable frequency reaches about 250 Hz. This suggests that many low-frequency tones aren't audible until the frequency of the variable tone reaches 250 Hz. Now the sound is detectable.

- As you continue to move your finger to the right, you cross the 10-phon contour at about 350 Hz and the 20-phon contour at about 950 Hz. This suggests that, as the frequency of the variable tone is increased within this range, your perception of its loudness increases as well.

- As the frequency of the tone is increased from 950 Hz to about 3,500 Hz, loudness stays fairly constant, a bit above 20 phons.

- Moving your finger across the abscissa farther, reflecting an increase in variable frequency from 3,500 Hz through 16,000 Hz, you cross the 10-phon contour at about 8,000 Hz, and the threshold of audibility curve, 0 phons, at about 10,000 Hz. This suggests that the loudness of the tone *decreases* from 3,500 Hz through about 10,000 Hz.

- As the frequency of the tone increases above 10,000 Hz, it is no longer audible.

This exercise demonstrates that, as a low-intensity pure tone steadily increases in frequency from very low to very high, our perception of its loudness changes.

Repeat the exercise, but now place the ruler horizontally across the figure connecting the ordinate axis markers corresponding to variable intensity of 60 dB SPL, which reflects a moderately intense stimulus. Again, slowly move your finger across the ruler's straight edge, mimicking the process of keeping the intensity of a pure tone constant while increasing frequency. Notice the contour lines you cross and at which frequencies. You should discover that this 60 dB SPL tone remains inaudible until about 60 Hz.

- As the frequency of the variable tone increases from 60 Hz to 400 Hz, five contours are crossed, suggesting significant loudness growth within a relatively narrow frequency range. The loudness of this tone grows from just detectable to 50 phons within this range.

- As frequency continues to increase, loudness appears to stay fairly constant, a bit above 50 phons, until about 4,000 Hz.
- Once we increase the frequency of the tone above 5,000 Hz, the magnitude of the phon contour lines crossed decreases, suggesting that the loudness decreases.
- By the time we reach 16,000 Hz, the tone is audible, but the loudness is less than 10 phons.

Repeat the exercise a final time. This time place your ruler horizontally across the ordinate at 110 dB SPL. Slowly move your finger along the straightedge across the abscissa from left to right.

- Pay attention to the loudness contours you cross as the frequency of the variable tone is increased from 20 Hz through 8,000 Hz. Notice that, within this frequency range, the contours crossed vary from 90 phons to about 100 phons. This suggests that the loudness of the tone, always audible, varies from a loudness of 90 phons to 100 phons throughout a wide range of pure tone frequencies.
- Above 8,000 Hz, the loudness decreases somewhat with a further increase in frequency, such that the loudness of this intense pure tone is 70 phons at 16,000 Hz.

The important point is that when the stimulus intensity is very high, our perception of its loudness doesn't change much with changes in stimulus frequency throughout the range of 20 Hz through 16,000 Hz.

The importance of Fletcher and Munson's work regarding the effect of frequency on loudness perception is that it depends on the original magnitude of the stimulus. For low- and moderate-intensity sounds, frequency has a significant effect on our perceived loudness; put another way, the loudness of the sound depends very much on its frequency. For example, very low frequency sounds may not even be audible at low or moderate intensities. Once the frequency of the sound is such that it's audible, loudness changes noticeably with further changes in frequency. This is not the case with high-intensity sounds. When a sound is presented at a very high intensity, loudness changes very little with changes in frequency. Put simply, *loud is loud*. Once sounds possessing very high intensities are judged as very loud, any change in their frequency won't affect loudness judgments much.

WHAT FLETCHER AND MUNSON TELL US ABOUT LOUDNESS GROWTH ACROSS FREQUENCY

Fletcher and Munson's study highlights another important concept regarding our perception of loudness, specifically how our perception of loudness changes as the intensity of a sound changes for lower- and higher-frequency tones. We know that as stimulus intensity is increased, our perception of loudness increases, but Fletcher and Munson provide additional evidence regarding how loudness increases as a function of stimulus frequency. In other words, how does the *growth of loudness,* with stimulus intensity compare across low- and high-frequency sounds? Is the growth of loudness the same for all pure tone frequencies?

In Figure 5-11, notice that, when the frequency of the variable is very low (for example, 20–50 Hz), the equal loudness contours are bunched together, compared to when the variable frequency is higher (such as 1,000 Hz). It appears that, once the frequency of the variable stimulus is above about 500 Hz, the equal loudness contours are more or less equally spaced apart. What does this observation imply regarding our loudness perception of these low-frequency sounds? This experimental evidence suggests that our perceptions of loudness growth with intensity for very low frequency sounds and for higher-frequency sounds are very different. Because the equal loudness contours are more closely spaced for very low frequency variable tones, loudness grows *faster* as stimulus intensity increases. For higher-frequency variable tones, loudness appears to grow more *slowly* with increase in stimulus intensity.

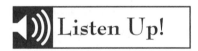 Listen Up!

PRACTICAL EXERCISE TO EXPLORE DIFFERENCES IN LOUDNESS GROWTH ACROSS FREQUENCY

Place a clear ruler *vertically* across Figure 5-11, connecting the ordinate axis markers corresponding to a variable frequency of 25 Hz. Now move your finger along the straightedge across the ordinate (variable intensity) from the bottom of the axis (0 dB SPL) through the top (140 dB SPL). Pay attention to the loudness contours you cross as you sweep your finger through the variable intensities. This exercise gives you an idea of how your loudness perception changes as you keep the *frequency* constant but steadily increase the *intensity* for this very low frequency tone.

- You should discover that the 25-Hz signal is below absolute threshold until its intensity reaches about 80 dB SPL. This suggests that these tones are inaudible until they reach an intensity of about 80 dB SPL. Now the sound is detectable.

- As you continue to move your finger up the intensity axis, you cross the phon contours rapidly, as the variable intensity is increased from 90 dB SPL through 110 dB SPL. This suggests that, as the intensity of the tone is increased within this range, your perception of its loudness increases significantly. In other words, when the intensity of a 25-Hz pure tone is increased from 90 dB SPL to 100 dB SPL, the loudness of the tone increases significantly from 10 phons to 50 phons. This suggests that a rather modest increase in intensity results in a large increase in loudness.

Compare this to when the variable frequency is equivalent to 2,000 Hz. Placing the clear ruler vertically across the figure, connect the ordinate axis markers corresponding to a variable frequency of 2,000 Hz. Now again move your finger along the straightedge across the ordinate from the bottom of the axis to the top, and pay attention to the loudness contours you cross as you sweep your finger through the range of variable intensities. Clearly, for this variable frequency, audibility occurs at a very low intensity, and loudness grows more gradually as the intensity increases.

Fletcher and Munson therefore provide additional information on the effect of the increase in stimulus intensity on loudness perception. Although for all sounds loudness increases as stimulus intensity increases, the growth of loudness with intensity depends on the *frequency* of the sound.

- For low-frequency sounds, loudness grows quickly as intensity increases, compared to mid- and high-frequency sounds. In other words, once a low-frequency sound becomes audible, its loudness increases significantly as its intensity is increased, even by a modest amount.

- Higher-frequency sounds, on the other hand, are audible at lower-intensity levels; we are more sensitive to the presence of these sounds. As we increase the intensity of these mid- and high-frequency sounds, the loudness increases modestly yet steadily, compared to their lower-frequency counterparts.

EXPLAINING LOUDNESS PERCEPTION

It is important to explain not only auditory perception and changes in our perceptions in response to the physical parameters of a signal, but also why our perceptions change as they do. Therefore, in addition to empirical evidence regarding our auditory perceptions related to loudness, hearing scientists also aim to provide models to help explain *why* our perceptions are the way they are. A **model** is a description or a theory to explain empirical evidence of behavior. To account for loudness growth as intensity increases and to explain why loudness growth is different for low- and high-frequency sounds, hearing scientists have developed the **excitation pattern**, which models neurological behavior at the level of the basilar membrane in the cochlea. It is a schematic representation of the total amount of neurological energy, or excitation, distributed across the entire length of the membrane. Recall that, moving from the base to the apex of the basilar membrane, the characteristic frequency of the individual nerve fibers innervating the organ of Corti change from high frequencies to progressively lower frequencies. When a simple stimulus like a pure tone enters the cochlea, a number of nerve fibers respond, generating a unique pattern of neurological activity. Fibers with characteristic frequencies very close to or equal to the frequency of the pure tone respond with the greatest amount of

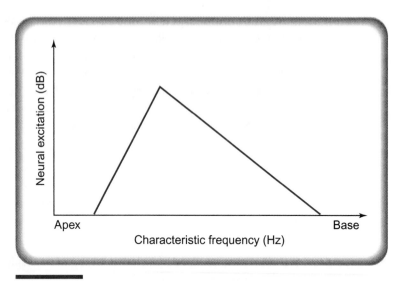

FIGURE 5-12 Excitation Pattern for a Moderately Intense Pure Tone.

neurological activity. As the characteristic frequency of the fibers is removed from the frequency of the pure tone (those positioned closer to the base or apex of the cochlea), the amount of neurological activity generated lessens.

Figure 5-12 presents an example of an excitation pattern for a moderately intense pure tone. The characteristic frequency of the individual nerve fibers innervating the basilar membrane, expressed in Hertz, is plotted on the abscissa. The excitation pattern enables us to view the basilar membrane as if it were being unrolled, where the characteristic frequencies of the individual fibers are displayed from low (on the left, representing the apex of the membrane) to high (on the right, representing the base of the membrane). The amount of neurological excitation, in decibels, is plotted on the ordinate.

In terms of the excitation pattern in response to a pure tone, the maximum amount of neurological activity occurs at a very specific point on the basilar membrane. At that point, the characteristic frequency of the innervating fiber equals the frequency of the stimulating pure tone. This is the frequency that this one fiber responds to *best*. Excitation *decreases* from the peak in two directions:

1. As the characteristic frequencies of the fibers become lower than the frequency of the pure tone, indicating that we are moving closer to the apex of the cochlea.

2. As the characteristic frequency of the fibers move higher than the frequency of the pure tone, indicating that we are moving closer to the base of the cochlea.

Notice also that the change in excitation is different for the low-frequency side of the excitation pattern, compared to the high-frequency side. The slope of

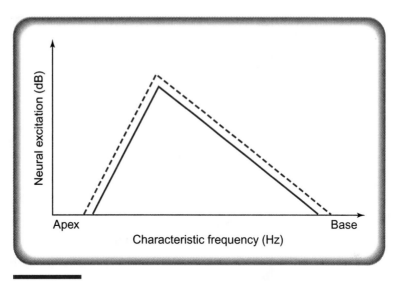

FIGURE 5-13 Two Excitation Patterns for a Pure Tone at Two Different Intensities: The dotted pattern reflects a slightly higher-intensity pure tone than the solid pattern.

the low-frequency side is *much steeper* than that of the high-frequency side due to the distinctive characteristics of the traveling wave response. Remember that the amplitude of the traveling wave grows somewhat gradually until the point of maximum excitation is reached. Once the amplitude of the traveling wave reaches its maximum, the response dampens quickly. Recall also that higher-frequency tones result in a maximum traveling wave amplitude near the base of the cochlea and that lower-frequency tones result in maximum traveling wave amplitude near the apex. Therefore, because more higher-frequency fibers are stimulated reaching the maximum peak of the traveling wave response, the slope on the high-frequency side of the excitation pattern is more gradual. Once the peak is reached and the traveling wave response dampens, the fibers corresponding to the apical end of the cochlea are not stimulated as much.

Figure 5-13 shows how the excitation pattern helps to explain why our loudness perception grows with the increase in stimulus intensity. Two excitation patterns are represented in response to two pure tones. The solid function represents the pattern provided by a pure tone presented at a moderate intensity. The dotted function represents the pattern provided by another pure tone, at the same frequency as the first but at a higher intensity. Notice that the overall characteristics of both excitation patterns are similar: The peaks of both responses occur at the same characteristic frequency, and the high-frequency slopes of both patterns are shallower than those on the low-frequency side.

What difference between these two patterns could the ear be using to determine that one pure tone is louder than the other? Clearly, the overall areas of

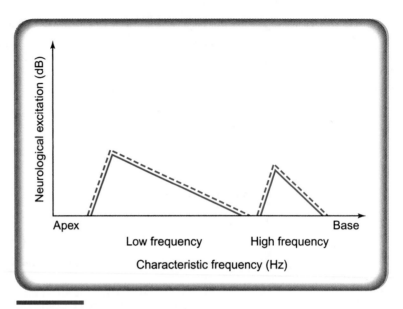

FIGURE 5-14 Difference in Loudness Growth, with Intensity, for Low-
and High-Frequency Pure Tones: The excitation patterns
are for two pure tone frequencies at two intensities. The
dotted patterns reflect slightly higher-intensity pure
tones than the solid patterns. (From Moore, 2003.)

the two patterns are different; the area of the dotted pattern is larger than that of
the solid pattern. Therefore, the stimulus corresponding to the higher-intensity
excitation pattern is recognized as louder, compared to the stimulus corresponding to the lower-intensity pattern.

Figure 5-14 illustrates how excitation patterns help explain why low-frequency
tones grow more quickly in loudness than higher-frequency tones as intensity
is raised (as Fletcher and Munson demonstrated). Four excitation patterns
are represented.

The *solid* patterns reflect two pure tones at moderate intensity levels: one
low frequency (on the left-hand side) and one high frequency (on the
right-hand side).

The *dashed* patterns reflect the changes in the excitation patterns for the same
two low- and high-frequency pure tones at slightly higher intensities.

As Fletcher and Munson determined, we judge the growth in loudness for
low-frequency tones greater than that for high-frequency tones. The excitation patterns represented in Figure 5-14 reflect this behavior. If we compare the increase in
the overall area of neurological stimulation from the lower-frequency pure tones,
as intensity is increased, to the change in overall area of neurological stimulation

from the higher-frequency patterns, clearly the greater increase in area occurs for the lower-frequency tones. The ear interprets the greater increase in excitation pattern area associated with the lower-frequency tones as a more significant increase in loudness.

Modeling our auditory perceptions based on excitation patterns in the cochlea does a good job of explaining the behaviors we have studied based on previous empirical studies on loudness. We will revisit excitation patterns when we explain other aspects of our normal auditory perceptions.

■ CHAPTER SUMMARY

We have covered many important concepts related to normal human loudness perception. After reading and studying this chapter, you should be able to:

- Provide a definition for the psychological perception of loudness.
- Explain the difference between physical parameters of sound and psychological perceptions to sound and why these differences are important to remember.
- Describe the relationship between sound intensity and loudness.
- Define an experimental paradigm and how this representation of the conditions of a listening experiment is helpful to beginning students of hearing science.
- Compare and contrast the two primary ways in which hearing scientists obtain loudness estimates from listeners: direct and indirect procedures.
- Explain how these procedures are similar and in what important ways they are different, providing an example of an experimental paradigm used for each procedure.
- Compare and contrast the two units of loudness estimation: the sone and the phon.
- Define an equal loudness contour, and describe how different equal loudness contours can and can't be compared.
- Compare and contrast the importance of stimulus frequency on loudness for low-, moderate-, and high-intensity sounds.
- Define growth of loudness as it relates to changes in stimulus intensity.
- Compare and contrast the growth of loudness, with stimulus intensity, for low-, moderate-, and high-frequency pure tones.
- Define the term "model" and explain why models are important to the study of hearing science, as well as what additional information they provide to students of hearing science.

- Define an excitation pattern and provide an example for a moderately intense pure tone, highlighting important characteristics.

- Describe how the concept of the excitation pattern explains the following perceptions related to loudness: increase in loudness with increase in stimulus intensity; the greater increase in loudness growth, in response to stimulus intensity, for low-frequency tones than for higher-frequency tones.

REFERENCES

Fletcher, H., and W. A. Munson. "Loudness, Its Definition, Measurement and Calculation." *Journal of the Acoustical Society of America* 5 (1933): 82–108.

Moore, B. C. J. "Pitch Perception." In *An Introduction to the Psychology of Hearing*, 5th ed., 158–193. San Diego, CA: Academic Press, 2003.

Sivian, L. J., and S. D. White. "On Minimum Audible Sound Fields." *Journal of the Acoustical Society of America* 4 (1933): 288–321.

Stevens, J. C., and E. Tulving. "Estimations of Loudness by a Group of Untrained Observers." *American Journal of Psychology* 70 (1957): 600–605.

6

INTENSITY DISCRIMINATION

LEARNING OBJECTIVES

The important concepts you will learn in this chapter are:

- Sensory discrimination and how it relates to stimulus intensity and the auditory system.

- The importance of auditory discrimination ability in hearing science.

- Amplitude modulation and primary auditory beats.

- Experimental studies of normal human intensity discrimination ability—old and new.

- The role of stimulus intensity in our ability to discriminate changes in stimulus intensity.

- The role of stimulus frequency in our ability to discriminate changes in stimulus intensity.

- The historical significance of Weber's fraction and Weber's law.

- The ability of Weber's law to adequately predict normal human differential sensitivity to intensity.

- The use of the excitation pattern as a model to explain our remarkable ability to discriminate changes in stimulus intensity.

KEY TERMS

Amplitude Modulation

ΔI

ΔS

Detection

Difference Limen (DL)

Differential Thresholds of Sensitivity

Discrimination

Discrimination Ability for Intensity

Discrimination Threshold

Just Noticeable Difference (jnd)

Method of Constant Stimuli

Primary Auditory Beats

Psychometric Function

Resolving Power

Saturation

Weber Fraction

Weber's Law

OVERVIEW

Regarding the hierarchy of auditory behavior, we have learned that the most fundamental level is detection. **Detection**, you may recall, is the ability to determine the presence of a sound. You don't have to be able to identify or label it, nor do you have to determine whether it is the same as or different from another sound. You only have to be able to detect its presence, relative to silence. In this chapter, we explore the next level of auditory processing: auditory discrimination. The word **discrimination** comes from the Latin *discriminare*, which means to "distinguish between." In terms of auditory behavior, discrimination is our ability to judge sounds as being the same or different. In other words, if we are presented with two sounds that are physically different along some acoustic parameter, can we perceive the difference? Do the sounds strike us as the same or different? In this chapter, we explore our **discrimination ability for intensity**, that is, how different do two sounds have to be in intensity for us to judge them as being different? Do the frequencies of the sounds influence our ability to discriminate their intensities? Does our ability to judge intensity differences depend on their presentation level or on loudness?

DISCRIMINATION THRESHOLDS: TERMINOLOGY AND RELEVANCE

Auditory discrimination ability is quantified in terms of a **discrimination threshold**, much as auditory sensitivity is quantified in relation to an absolute threshold. Thresholds of discrimination go by a variety of names.

- Sometimes they are referred to as **difference limens (DLs)**. "Limen" is another name for threshold. A difference limen is a threshold related to the smallest difference along some stimulus dimension that can just be detected.

- Another synonymous term is the **just noticeable difference (jnd)**.

- Finally, discrimination thresholds may be represented as ΔS, where "Δ" is the Greek symbol for change, and "S" represents the acoustic stimulus parameter of interest.

- **Differential thresholds of sensitivity**, another generic term for discrimination thresholds, may be measured across a number of different stimulus parameters related to all of our senses. Because we are concerned with auditory perceptions, we will limit the discussion to discrimination ability as it relates to the acoustic variable of intensity.

Whichever term is used, they all represent the same concept.

Discrimination ability for intensity is important to understand because it represents an important step in the hierarchy of auditory behavior. In defining the limits of auditory discrimination, we are able to describe the **resolving power** of the auditory system: How sensitive are we to changes in some particular dimension of a sound? In the case of intensity, if we discover that we are able to detect relatively small changes in sound intensity with a fairly high degree of accuracy, then we describe our resolving power for intensity as high or good. On the other hand, if we require substantially large differences in the intensity between two sounds to judge them as being different, then we describe our resolving power for intensity as low or poor. Auditory discrimination thresholds allow us to define our resolution ability for the physical parameters of a sound.

■ EXPERIMENTAL MEASUREMENTS OF NORMAL AUDITORY INTENSITY DISCRIMINATION

The most often cited published report defining the limits of human auditory discrimination threshold for intensity is a study performed at Bell Laboratories by R. R. Riesz in 1928. The ingenious experimental paradigm used by Riesz to investigate normal human differential sensitivity for intensity is not the typical paradigm used today. However, it highlights an unusual auditory perception that we experience when two pure tones of slightly different frequencies are mixed and delivered to the auditory system. This auditory perception is termed **primary auditory beats**, which is the psychological perception a listener experiences when presented with two mixed pure tones of slightly different frequencies.

Figure 6-1 illustrates the physical interaction of two such pure tones. In the figure, the waveforms of two pure tones with slightly different frequencies are represented in the top and middle panels. The period (T) of the first waveform is slightly longer than that of the second waveform. If a pure tone's period is inversely related to its frequency, the frequency of the pure tone waveform in the top panel (T_1) is lower than the frequency of the pure tone waveform in the middle panel (T_2). Keep in mind that the differences in the period and frequency between these two pure tones are very small. Notice that the amplitudes of the two pure tones are identical and equal to 1 unit.

The bottom waveform represents the result when the two original pure tones are physically combined, or mixed. The combination of these two pure tones—of slightly different frequencies and identical intensities—results in a complex periodic waveform. The amplitude of the combined waveform changes over time from *almost* complete summation (2 units) to *almost* complete cancellation (0 units). Over a longer period of time, the amplitude of the resulting waveform will wax and wane periodically between these two extremes. In fact, the frequency with which the amplitude waxes and wanes, from its minimum value to its maximum value, equals the difference in frequency between the two original pure tones. For example, if the first pure tone has a frequency of 1,000 Hz and is combined with a second pure tone with a frequency of 1,003 Hz, the combined waveform

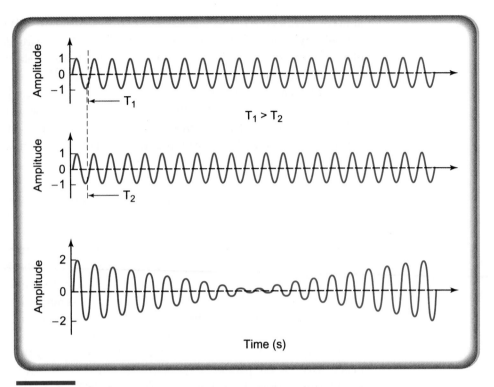

FIGURE 6-1 **Waveforms of Pure Tones Producing Amplitude Modulation and the Perception of Beats:** The top two waveforms illustrate two pure tones with periods T_1 and T_2. The period of waveform T_1 is lightly longer than that of waveform T_2. The bottom waveform is the complex, periodic, amplitude-modulated stimulus resulting from the physical combination of waveforms T_1 and T_2.

would cycle through the maximum and minimum excursions in amplitude three times per second. The cyclical change in the physical amplitude of the combined waveform is referred to as **amplitude modulation.** When we listen to the combined waveform, we detect the modulation in amplitude as auditory beats. In other words, we perceive a pure tone changing in loudness over time.

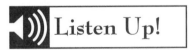

AMPLITUDE MODULATION AND SIGNAL TRANSMISSION

You may already be familiar with the term "amplitude modulation" as it applies to radio transmissions. Most radio receivers are able to pick up radio transmissions by either amplitude modulation (AM) or frequency modulation (FM), both of which are techniques used to transmit information via radio waves. Amplitude modulation as it applies to primary auditory beats is not the same as amplitude modulation as it relates to radio transmission. With respect to primary auditory beats, amplitude modulation refers to the physical changes of the envelope of a complex periodic waveform as a function of time. It has nothing to do with radio transmission.

Riesz used the perception of primary beats to measure intensity discrimination thresholds. He mixed and delivered the output, monoaurally, of two pure tone oscillators to 12 normal-hearing subjects. The difference in frequency between the two oscillators was always 3 Hz. In this way, the mixed signal delivered to the listeners was an amplitude-modulated periodic complex tone. The intensity of one oscillator was adjusted to a predetermined level above the subjects' threshold. The intensity of the second oscillator was set to a level well below the intensity of the first oscillator.

As the subjects listened to the mixed output from these two oscillators, Riesz gradually increased the intensity of the second oscillator until the listener signaled the presence of beats. As a result, at the start of the experimental trial, when the intensity of the second oscillator was much less than the first, the listeners perceived a steady pure tone. As the intensity of the second oscillator increased, so did the amplitude modulation of the combined output. Once the amplitude modulation became significant enough to be noticeable to the listener—the point at which the output tone changed from steady to wavering (beats)—the procedure was stopped, and the intensities of the first and second oscillators were recorded.

The intensity recorded for the second oscillator represented the lowest intensity for beats to just become noticeable. If the intensity of the second oscillator was adjusted to just below the recorded level, the tone would be steady (no beats), and if the intensity of the second tone was increased above the recorded level, the tone would waver (beats). Using a complex formula involving the recorded intensities of the two oscillators, Riesz was able to calculate the difference limen, in dB, for the characteristics of the listening condition, determined by the frequency and the intensity of the first oscillator.

Riesz performed this procedure using five different pure tone frequencies, from 35 Hz through 10,000 Hz, and a number of different pure tone intensities, from near-threshold to 90 dB higher. His results allow us to understand the resolving power of the auditory system for intensity as a function of frequency and as a function of intensity.

ANOTHER METHOD FOR ESTIMATING INTENSITY DISCRIMINATION THRESHOLDS

Riesz's experimental results concerning our differential sensitivity for intensity have been replicated numerous times. While these replication studies demonstrate the same conclusions reported by Riesz nearly 100 years ago, the experimental procedure used by more recent studies is very different from his. This procedure is very old but can be modified to make use of modern technology. The **method of constant stimuli** is an experimental procedure used to measure thresholds of discrimination including intensity discrimination thresholds. It is one of several traditional psychophysical experimental procedures that hearing scientists employ and the traditional psychophysical procedure frequently used to assess auditory differential sensitivity.

Let's explore the characteristics of the method of constant stimuli using a hypothetical example of an auditory experiment designed to measure the intensity difference limen for a 1,000-Hz pure tone moderately above threshold. The experimental paradigm for such an investigation is illustrated in Figure 6-2. Two stimuli, standard and variable, are presented to a listener.

1. The *standard stimulus* reflects the conditions in which the experimenter is interested in estimating differential sensitivity. In this example, the standard stimulus is a 1,000-Hz pure tone presented at 50 dB SL. The frequency and the intensity of the standard remain the same throughout the experiment.

2. The *variable stimulus* is also a 1,000-Hz pure tone. Because the experimenter is interested in measuring *differential sensitivity for intensity* (not frequency), the frequency of the variable stimulus remains equal to the standard (1,000 Hz) throughout the experiment. The intensity of the variable stimulus is represented in terms of five values that are preselected by the experimenter.

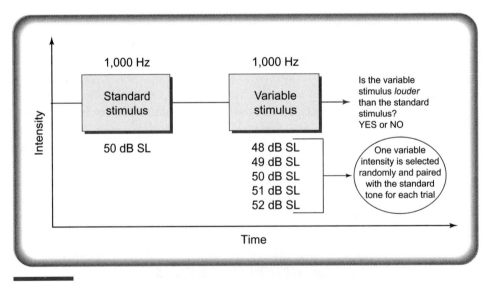

FIGURE 6-2 Experimental Paradigm of the Method of Constant Stimuli: The example shows the stimulus parameters used to estimate the intensity discrimination threshold of a listener at 1,000 Hz, 50 dB SL.

Two variable intensity values are below the intensity of the standard, two are higher, and one is equal to the standard. The method of constant stimuli is so named because a small number of preselected *constant* variables, usually five or seven, are ultimately paired with the standard.

In this experimental paradigm, each of the five variable stimuli is randomly paired with the standard stimulus, ultimately many times throughout the procedure. Let's imagine that the experimenter decides to pair each variable stimulus 100 times with the standard. This will result in a total of 500 listening trials. Keep in mind that, for any one trial during the procedure, the intensity of the variable stimulus is randomly selected from the five values preselected by the experimenter.

For each stimulus pair presented, the listener's task is to decide whether the variable stimulus is louder or softer than the standard. The experimenter decides beforehand whether the variable is to be judged always louder or always softer than the standard. In our example, the experimenter has the listener judging whether the variable is louder. This is a two-alternative forced-choice procedure. For each trial, the listener must vote either yes or no as to whether the second pure tone is louder than the first. Even if the tones seem equal in loudness, the listener must answer yes or no. For each trial, the experimenter records the yes or the no vote and continues until the total number of listening trials is completed.

Table 6-1 Illustrates a summary of the results across the 500 trials of our hypothetical study. In this table, each of the five variable intensities is shown with the total number of yes votes recorded for the 100 trials in which the variable intensity was paired with the standard stimulus.

TABLE 6-1 Hypothetical Results of an Intensity Discrimination Study Using the Method of Constant Stimuli.

Intensity of the Variable Stimulus (dB SL)	Number of Times the Variable Stimulus Was Judged Louder Than the Standard Stimulus	Total Number of Times the Variable Stimulus Intensity Was Paired with the Standard Stimulus	Percentage of Times the Variable Stimulus Was Judged Louder Than the Standard (%)
48	10	100	10
49	30	100	30
50	60	100	60
51	80	100	80
52	95	100	95

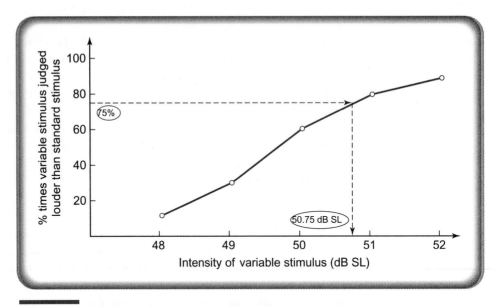

FIGURE 6-3 Psychometric Function Generated from Table 6-1: Subject's performance is plotted as a function of variable stimulus intensity. The arrows illustrate the intensity of the variable stimulus corresponding to 75 percent performance. The standard stimulus is a 1,000-Hz pure tone, 50 dB SL.

From this table, the experimenter generates a **psychometric function** (illustrated in Figure 6-3), which plots the occurrence of an auditory perception as a function of a physical stimulus parameter. In this case, the experimenter plots the percentage of times the listener judged the variable tone louder than the standard (a yes vote) as a function of the five intensity levels of the variable tone. The experimenter could easily have decided to represent the psychometric function in terms of the percentage of times the listener judged the variable tone softer than the standard (a no vote) as a function of the variable intensity. In either case, the estimate of differential sensitivity would ultimately be the same. In our example, however, the experimenter decided to represent the percentage of yes votes: the percentage of times that each level of the variable tone was judged louder than the standard.

To estimate the intensity difference limen from our hypothetical experiment, the experimenter extrapolates the intensity of the variable stimulus corresponding to 75 percent performance. In other words, the question is, from the psychometric function generated, which variable intensity corresponds to the listener's judgment that the loudness of the variable tone is louder than the standard tone 75 percent of the time? More often than not, the 75 percent performance point does not exactly correspond to one of the preselected levels of the variable, as in our hypothetical experiment. Rather, the 75 percent performance is estimated, or interpolated, from the psychometric function.

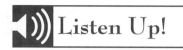 Listen Up!

WHY IS THE PERFORMANCE CRITERION FOR DIFFERENTIAL THRESHOLDS SET AT 75 PERCENT?

Differential thresholds of sensitivity are typically estimated using a 75 percent performance criterion, even though absolute thresholds (thresholds of detection) are determined using a 50 percent performance criterion. Why aren't the criteria the same? A performance criterion set at 50 percent, particularly when only two alternatives exist, represents chance performance. By using a 50 percent performance criterion (instead of listening to the two stimuli and making judgments concerning relative loudness), the listener might just as well flip a coin to decide whether the second tone is louder than the first. Hearing scientists believe that a 50 percent criterion for estimating thresholds of discrimination is too lax; it is too close to a chance performance level. On the other hand, selecting a 100 percent performance criterion is too stringent because we are attempting to estimate a *threshold* of auditory perception. The 75 percent performance criterion, however, represents the midpoint between the too lax 50 percent performance and the too stringent 100 percent performance criterion.

With respect to our hypothetical experiment, Figure 6-3 shows that the intensity of the variable stimulus corresponding to 75 percent performance is 50.75 dB SL. Theoretically, if a 1,000-Hz, 50-dB SL standard is paired with a 1,000-Hz, 50.75-dB SL variable, this listener judges the second stimulus (variable) as louder than the first three times out of four.

To measure the difference limen (ΔI), we take the difference between the two intensities, calculated using the following expression:

$$\Delta I = I(\text{std}) - I(\text{var})$$

where $I(\text{std})$ is the intensity of the standard stimulus and $I(\text{var})$ is the intensity of the variable stimulus at 75 percent performance. The absolute value of this difference is used to allow for judgments of loudness as louder or softer than the standard.

For our hypothetical experiment, the difference between the intensity of the standard and the intensity of the variable at 75 percent performance is 0.75 dB. Therefore, the intensity difference limen for this listener at 1,000 Hz, 50 dB above absolute threshold is 0.75 dB. Two 1,000-Hz pure tones, presented to this listener around 50 dB SL and having an intensity difference *exceeding* 0.75 dB, will always be judged as being *different*. On the other hand, if these same two pure tones are presented to this listener with an intensity difference *less than* 0.75 dB, they will always be judged as being the *same*.

The intensity difference limen of 0.75 dB corresponds to the smallest difference in intensity that the listener can just detect, given the frequency and intensity characteristics of the standard stimulus.

- Intensity differences greater than this amount correspond to the listener's *always* perceiving the difference between the two sounds.

- Intensity differences less than this value correspond to the listener's *never* perceiving the difference between the two sounds.

This is an important distinction because, when the intensity difference between two sounds is less than the jnd, the physical difference between the two sounds is still present, albeit small. In our hypothetical experiment, objectively, we can measure the physical intensity difference between, say, a 1,000-Hz, 50-dB SL standard pure tone and a 1,000-Hz, 50.5-dB SL variable pure tone. Our listener, however, cannot perceive the physical difference in intensity between these two tones because the intensity difference is less than the listener's differential sensitivity threshold. These two pure tones sound exactly the same to the listener. This is another good example of the distinction between the measurement of physical sound parameters and our subjective measurements of their perceptions.

■ NORMAL HUMAN AUDITORY DIFFERENTIAL THRESHOLDS FOR INTENSITY

The results reported by Riesz, shown in Figure 6-4, have been corroborated by more recent investigations concerning differential thresholds of intensity (Jesteadt, Wier, and Green, 1977; Viemeister, 1972). Figure 6-4 plots the intensity differential threshold (ΔI) as a function of intensity for the five different pure tone frequencies investigated by Riesz. In the experimental context of the method of constant stimuli, the independent variables represented in the figure reflect the intensity and the frequency of the standard stimulus.

Before we begin to explore what we can learn from Riesz's study regarding the role of frequency and intensity on our ability to differentiate intensity, we need to understand the meaning behind the metric used for these estimates, namely ΔI. Recall that ΔI

- Reflects the *smallest* intensity difference between two sounds that the listener can just notice.

- Provides an estimate of the magnitude of our *resolving power* for intensity.

In other words:

- When ΔI is relatively large, our ability to resolve or discriminate signals along the dimension of intensity is relatively poor. We need a larger difference between the intensity of two sounds to perceive them as being different.

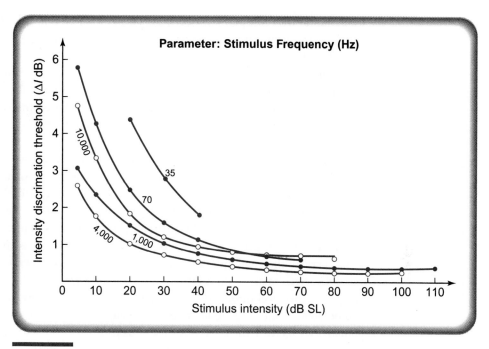

FIGURE 6-4 Differential Thresholds for Intensity as a Function of Pure Tone Intensity and Frequency. (After Riesz, 1928.)

- When ΔI is estimated to be relatively small, our resolution ability for intensity is relatively good. We can perceive rather small physical differences in intensity between two sounds and recognize them as being different.

As we review Riesz's findings, keep in mind that, as ΔI increases, our ability to resolve sounds along the intensity continuum becomes poorer. Likewise, as the magnitude of ΔI decreases, our resolving power improves.

THE ROLE OF INTENSITY ON DIFFERENTIAL SENSITIVITY FOR INTENSITY

In Figure 6-4, for all of the variable frequencies represented, a similar trend is evident regarding the magnitude of ΔI as the intensity of the standard tone is increased. For tones characterized by intensities moderately above threshold (40 dB SL), ΔI is relatively low, about 1 dB. As the intensity of the tones are increased to levels well above threshold, up to 100 dB SL or more, ΔI decreases slightly but remains fairly constant at 0.5–1 dB throughout the range. Notice that the functions reflecting the parameter of the graph (standard tone frequency) are very close together throughout this range. So it appears that, for moderately intense tones, ΔI is relatively small. As the intensity of the tones increase further, ΔI decreases a little bit more but for the most part stays constant between 0.5 dB and 1 dB, throughout a very broad range of stimulus intensities.

An entirely different trend is evident for stimulus intensities below 40 dB SL. As the intensity of the standard tones drops below about 40 dB SL, the magnitude of ΔI increases, especially for tones just slightly above threshold (20 dB SL or less). So it appears from these results that intensity discrimination thresholds for soft sounds are relatively large and become larger as the intensity of the sounds are reduced, approaching detection thresholds.

Hearing scientists interpret these experimental results in the following way. Our ability to discriminate intensity differences between two sounds very much depends on their *audibility*. For example, when sounds are very audible, at 40 dB SL or so, intensity discrimination thresholds are relatively small. (Small values of ΔI mean that we can reliably perceive small physical differences in intensity between sounds, and they suggest that our resolving power for intensity is good.) Further, as we increase the audibility of sounds from these moderate levels to louder levels, differential intensity threshold decreases modestly, to less than 0.05 dB, and remains at this level throughout the upper limits of the dynamic range. For very audible sounds, then, our ability to detect small differences in the intensity is very good. As we increase the audibility of sounds further (creating loud sounds), our discrimination ability improves slightly and remains very good over a large range of intensities. We are very sensitive to changes in stimulus intensity for sounds that are moderately loud, loud, and very loud.

Soft sounds paint an entirely different picture. To discriminate soft sounds accurately, we require larger intensity differences. Our resolving power for intensity for these sounds is poorer than that for louder sounds. Further, as soft sounds become less audible, approaching the intensity levels we need to detect them, we also need larger physical differences in intensity to judge them as being different. Our resolving power becomes poorer as we approach the absolute threshold. Clearly, the sound's intensity influences our intensity discrimination ability much more than in the case of moderately loud and loud sounds. In conclusion, the role of intensity on our differential sensitivity is significant for soft sounds, but not for moderately loud and loud sounds.

THE ROLE OF FREQUENCY ON DIFFERENTIAL SENSITIVITY FOR INTENSITY

Look at the pattern of the five functions plotted in Figure 6-4, reflecting the five pure tone frequencies investigated by Riesz. For the most part, they appear to be somewhat parallel, suggesting that the effects of stimulus intensity on intensity discrimination thresholds are the same regardless of the pure tone's frequency. For low-frequency, mid-frequency, and high-frequency sounds, our discrimination ability for intensity is relatively poor for soft sounds, especially those very close to threshold, and it improves significantly once the tones become moderately loud.

For moderately loud and loud sounds, our discrimination ability for intensity remains very good and constant, regardless of the sound's frequency. Frequency does not appear to have much influence on the overall trends discussed so far.

This is not to say, however, that frequency plays no role in determining differential thresholds for intensity. Frequency is an important parameter influencing our ability to discriminate intensity differences between sounds, especially soft sounds. In Figure 6-4, the functions reflecting the different pure tone frequencies become more widely spaced as the intensity of the sounds approach threshold. Note particularly the ordering of the frequencies at the low-intensity levels: the pure tone frequencies that yield the lowest values of ΔI and those that correspond to the highest values. We see that the 4,000-Hz pure tone yields the lowest values of ΔI, followed by 1,000 Hz and 10,000 Hz. The two lower pure tone frequencies, 70 Hz and 35 Hz, correspond to the highest relative magnitude for ΔI. Keeping in mind the rule for interpreting ΔI magnitude, this observation suggests that, for soft sounds:

- Our ability to discriminate changes in intensity is best for mid-frequency sounds.

- Our differential sensitivity for intensity is poorest for very low frequency sounds.

- High-frequency sounds fall in the middle of these two extremes.

Once the presentation level of the tones increases, the relative differences in ΔI seen for low-, mid-, and high-frequency sounds disappear. The functions are very close together at these intensities.

What is it about the mid-frequency tones that so influences our differential sensitivity for intensity? Why is it easier to discriminate intensity differences for these sounds, compared to high- and low-frequency sounds, especially when they are just audible? Hearing scientists think the answer is related to our detection ability, as explained in Chapter 4. In terms of absolute sensitivity (detection), we are most sensitive to the presence of sounds with frequencies between 1,000 Hz and 5,000 Hz, the same frequencies as those related to our best ability to resolve intensity. It should come as no surprise that the pure tone frequencies that our auditory system is most sensitive to regarding absolute sensitivity are those corresponding to our best differential sensitivity for intensity.

In summary, the role of frequency on our ability to discriminate the intensity differences between two pure tones depends on the overall loudness of the tones, much like the effect of intensity on this ability. Specifically, frequency does not seem to play much of a role in determining our relative ability to discriminate intensity differences between two sounds if the sounds are moderately loud or loud. ΔI thresholds are low and very similar for all pure tone frequencies within this range. Frequency appears to have a much larger influence in determining our discrimination ability for intensity for soft sounds, especially those very close to threshold. For these sounds, frequencies that correspond to our most sensitive regions, in terms of detection, also suggest our best ability in terms of differential sensitivity to intensity. Frequencies that fall outside of our most sensitive region correspond to a poorer ability to distinguish intensity.

■ SCIENTIFIC INTEREST IN DIFFERENTIAL SENSITIVITY

In the early nineteenth century, the scientific study of psychophysics was in its infancy. Scientists were just beginning to explore the limits of perception and the relationship of our perceptions to physical stimulation. These explorations involved a number of our human senses and were not limited to hearing.

In the early 1800s, a German anatomist and physiologist by the name of Ernst Heinrich Weber published the results of a series of studies related to differential thresholds regarding the sense of touch. Weber was interested in the differential sensitivity of weight. If a subject is holding a 50-lb weight, what is the smallest increase in weight that was just noticeable? From these investigations, Weber found an interesting and ultimately important relationship between the jnd for the perceived weight of an object and its original weight: The change in a stimulus that is just noticeable is a constant ratio of the original stimulus.

A student of Weber by the name of Gustav Theodor Fechner went on to develop this relationship. Fechner, a bit of a philosopher, was convinced that the relationship between differential sensitivity and original stimulus strength was a constant value, unifying all of our senses. He postulated this relationship as **Weber's law,** in honor of his mentor, and expressed it as

$$\frac{\Delta S}{S} = \text{constant}$$

where ΔS = the discrimination threshold and S = the magnitude of the stimulus. In other words, the differential sensitivity threshold related to a particular perception is a constant proportion of its original stimulus magnitude ($\Delta S/S$). This equation suggests the following:

- As the magnitude of the original stimulus *increases,* differential sensitivity increases.

- As the magnitude of the original stimulus *decreases,* differential sensitivity decreases.

Also:

- As the difference limen (ΔS) *increases,* our ability to perceive changes in the stimulus gets poorer.

- As the difference limen *decreases,* our ability to perceive changes to the stimulus gets better.

The expression $\Delta S/S$ is known as the **Weber fraction,** and the idea that this expression remains constant throughout a range of stimulus magnitudes is known as Weber's law. In the case of the auditory system, if Weber's law holds true, we should see empirical evidence suggesting that, as the intensity of a sound increases, ΔI increases proportionately, that is, our differential sensitivity becomes poorer. Likewise, as sound intensity decreases, ΔI should decrease as well, suggesting that our differential sensitivity improves.

Figure 6-4 shows that the experimental evidence does not support Weber's law. In that figure, we see that, for a very wide range of stimulus intensities, our differential threshold for intensity remains constant, whereas Weber's law predicts steadily increasing values of ΔI as stimulus intensity increases.

Further evidence of the "near miss" of Weber's law is illustrated in Figure 6-5, which presents a compilation of studies measuring intensity discrimination thresholds for a 1,000-Hz pure tone (Campbell and Lasky, 1967; Harris, 1952, 1963; Luce and Green, 1974; McGill and Goldberg, 1968; Riesz, 1928). In this figure, the Weber fraction for auditory intensity $(\Delta I/I)$ is plotted as a function of stimulus intensity. Clearly, in general, the Weber fraction decreases as stimulus intensity increases, just as we would expect based on the empirical evidence reported by Riesz but contrary to the consistency theorized by Fechner many years ago, at least for pure tones. Empirical evidence from experiments using more complex stimuli, however, suggests that Weber's law is more accurate in predicting our differential sensitivity for intensity (Miller, 1947).

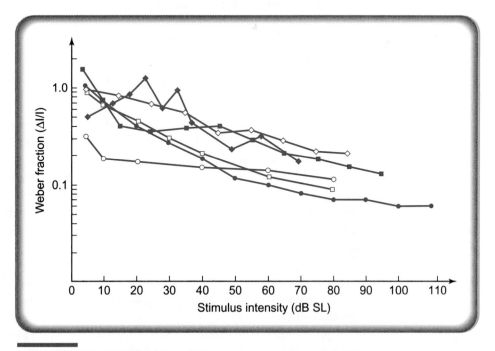

FIGURE 6-5 **Weber Fraction for Intensity as a Function of Stimulus Intensity: The figure represents a compilation of a number of recent studies reporting differential thresholds for pure tones of varying intensities. (After Green, 1976.)**

In summary, our differential sensitivity regarding sound intensity is much better than what Weber's law predicts. Weber's law significantly *underestimates* our remarkable ability to discriminate very small intensity differences over a very broad range of stimulus intensity. Our auditory system is exquisitely sensitive to changes in sound intensity.

The ear's intensity-resolving power is extremely important. The primary function of the auditory system is to detect and discriminate speech and, ultimately, to deliver this complex auditory stimulus to the brain in a recognizable form. Speech is a very complex auditory stimulus that is characterized, in part, by changes in intensity over time. Sometimes the changes in intensity are small, yet they carry powerful and important phonemic information. As a case in point, within the English language *fricatives* are an important class of consonants. These sounds are characterized by long intervals of noise produced by constriction at some point in the vocal tract. A special class of fricatives that includes the phonemes /s/, /z/, and /sh/ is known as *sibilants*, has long been distinguished from other fricatives like /f/, /v/, /th/, and /h/. During the production of sibilants, their overall intensity is greater than that for other fricatives (Kent and Read, 1992), and this intensity difference has been assumed to be an important perceptual cue for these speech sounds, although it is likely not the only acoustic cue we use for accurate identification of these consonants (Behrens and Blumstein, 1988). In any event, being able to recognize intensity differences among certain speech sounds has a tremendous effect on our ability to correctly discriminate, recognize, and comprehend important phonemic distinctions in our language.

A MODEL TO EXPLAIN OUR DIFFERENTIAL SENSITIVITY FOR INTENSITY

Hearing scientists use the excitation pattern model to explain our ability to maintain an extraordinary intensity discrimination performance throughout a very large range of stimulus intensities. Figure 6-6 illustrates the excitation pattern arising from two pure tones of the same frequency at slightly different intensity levels. The solid pattern reflects the lower presentation level, and the dashed pattern reflects a slightly higher presentation level (1–2 dB). This is a large enough difference in intensity for a listener to reliably distinguish the two tones (i.e., the intensity difference is larger than ΔI).

The excitation patterns of the two pure tones in Figure 6-6 look a little different than those illustrated in Chapter 5 (see Figure 5-12). The patterns in Figure 6-6 are characterized by a flat top. In other words, the amount of neurological excitation is high and constant throughout a finite frequency range surrounding the frequency of the pure tone. The excitation patterns in Chapter 5 reflected pure tones with a single characteristic frequency corresponding to maximum neurological excitation. As the characteristic frequency moved above or below the frequency of the pure

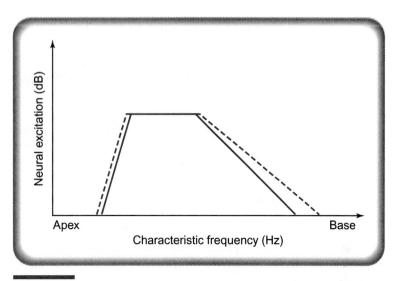

FIGURE 6-6 Excitation Patterns of Two Moderately Intense Pure Tones Differing Slightly in Intensity: The dashed line reflects a slightly higher intensity pure tone than the solid line.

tone, the amount of excitation dropped (a triangular pattern). The different pattern in Figure 6-6 is due to the presentation levels of the pure tones. The intensities of the two pure tones are much higher than those of the pure tone in Figure 5-12. They are so much higher, in fact, that the single-fiber neurons with characteristic frequencies somewhat above and below the stimulating pure tone frequency are saturated. **Saturation** occurs when the presentation level of a stimulus is high enough to drive the neurological activity of the fiber to its maximum level. Once an auditory nerve fiber reaches saturation, any additional increase in stimulus intensity does not result in an increase in neurological activity. The presentation levels of the two pure tones represented in Figure 6-6 are at levels high enough to saturate the single neurons with characteristic frequencies near the frequency of the pure tone—hence the flat tops. In fact, the presentation levels resulting in saturation are relatively modest, on the order of 40–50 dB above threshold. If Figure 6-6 illustrates the excitation pattern of two pure tones at presentation levels of, say, 80 dB SL and 82 dB SL, clearly these levels are much above the saturation levels for many of the single fibers near the frequency of the pure tone.

That said, what cues might the ear use to decide that the presentation levels of the two pure tones illustrated in Figure 6-6 are different? Clearly, the saturated fibers do not provide additional information as the intensity of the pure tone is raised a few decibels. Fibers with characteristic frequencies well below the frequency of the stimulating tone (not in saturation) also don't provide much information. The low-frequency slopes of the two patterns are the same. What does change noticeably is the slope of the *high-frequency side* of the excitation patterns. Notice that, as the presentation level of the pure tone is increased, the high-frequency side of the higher-intensity excitation pattern is noticeably shallower than the lower-intensity pattern. Scientists believe that the ear easily recognizes the change in slope on the high-frequency side of the two excitation patterns and senses that they are different. Therefore, we perceive the small physical change in the intensity of the two pure tones and can easily discriminate them, thereby explaining our phenomenal ability to distinguish small changes in presentation level, especially for moderate and high-intensity sounds.

■ CHAPTER SUMMARY

We have covered many important concepts related to normal human differential thresholds of sensitivity regarding stimulus intensity. After reading and studying this chapter, you should be able to do the following:

- Define auditory discrimination, explain how it is different from auditory detection, and identify its place in the hierarchy of auditory behavior.

- List the various terms that hearing scientists use to represent auditory discrimination and explain why auditory discrimination ability is important for us to describe and understand.

- Define the physical concept of amplitude modulation and how it relates to the perception of primary auditory beats.

- Outline Riesz's experimental paradigm for measuring normal human auditory discrimination thresholds.

- Outline the psychophysical procedure called the method of constant stimuli, as it is used to measure auditory discrimination thresholds.

- Calculate the auditory discrimination threshold from a psychometric function generated from a listener.

- Describe the role of stimulus intensity on our ability to discriminate intensity for soft, moderate, and loud pure tones.

- Describe the role of stimulus frequency on our ability to discriminate intensity for soft, moderate, and loud pure tones.

- Define Weber's fraction and Weber's law as they relate to sensory discrimination beyond the auditory system.

- Describe the ability of Weber's law to predict auditory intensity discrimination ability and explain how the empirical evidence from Riesz and others supports your statements regarding the accuracy of Weber's law in predicting differential sensitivity for stimulus intensity.

- Explain the importance of good auditory intensity discrimination as it relates to speech perception and provide an example.

- Describe the use of the excitation pattern as an adequate model to explain our extraordinary intensity discrimination ability over a very broad range of stimulus intensities.

■ REFERENCES

Behrens, S. and S. E. Blumstein. "On the Role of the Amplitude of the Fricative Noise in the Perception of Place of Articulation in Voiceless Fricative Consonants." *Journal of the Acoustical Society of America* 84 (1988): 861–867.

Campbell, R. A. and E. Z. Lasky. "Masker Level and Sinusoidal Signal Detection." *Journal of the Acoustical Society of America* 42 (1967): 972–976.

Green, D. M. *An Introduction to Hearing.* Mahwah, NJ: Lawrence Erlbaum Associates, 1976.

Harris, J. D. "Pitch Discrimination." *Journal of the Acoustical Society of America* 24 (1952): 750–755.

Harris, J. D. "Loudness Discrimination." *Journal of Speech and Hearing Disorders.* Monograph Supplement II, 1963.

Jesteadt, W., C. C. Wier, and D. M. Green. "Intensity Discrimination as a Function of Frequency and Sensation Level." *Journal of the Acoustical Society of America* 61 (1977): 169–177.

Kent, R. D. and C. Read. "The Acoustic Characteristics of Consonants." In *The Acoustic Analysis of Speech,* 105–144. San Diego, CA: Singular Publishing Group, 1992.

Luce, R. D. and D. M. Green. "Neural Coding and Psychophysical Discrimination Data." *Journal of the Acoustical Society of America* 56 (1974): 1554–1564.

McGill, W. J. and J. P. Goldberg. "Pure-Tone Intensity Discrimination and Energy Detection." *Journal of the Acoustical Society of America* 44 (1968): 576–581.

Miller, G. A. "Sensitivity to Changes in the Intensity of White Noise and Its Relation to Masking and Loudness." *Journal of the Acoustical Society of America* 19 (1974): 609–619.

Riesz, R. R. "Differential Sensitivity of the Ear for Pure Tones." *Physics Review* 31 (1928): 867–875.

Viemeister, N. F. "Intensity Discrimination of Pulsed Sinusoids: The Effects of Filtered Noise." *Journal of the Acoustical Society of America* 51 (1972): 1265–1269.

▪ FREQUENCY AS AN IMPORTANT STIMULUS VARIABLE TO AUDITORY PERCEPTION

As we explored the important role that stimulus intensity plays in our auditory perceptions, we learned much about the kinds of perceptions that hearing scientists are interested in studying. For example, the broad area of auditory perception can be narrowed to questions regarding sensitivity, discrimination, and our psychological experience with sound. We also introduced some of the traditional psychophysical procedures that hearing scientists employ to measure these auditory perceptions, including the method of constant stimuli for measuring auditory discrimination and the loudness balance procedure for loudness estimation. As we turn to the stimulus parameter of frequency, we will see many parallels in terms of the kinds of perceptions and abilities, with respect to frequency, that have interested hearing scientists over the last century. In addition, many of the experiments discussed in this section use experimental methods similar to those in the previous section. The detail provided on these psychophysical methods, as they relate to frequency, is less; so you may want to revisit previous chapters in the intensity section to refresh your memory. As we will see, the experimental questions and methods regarding the role of frequency on auditory perception very much parallel those we have discussed previously regarding stimulus intensity.

Frequency is a very important stimulus parameter in our auditory perceptions. We have already discovered that the frequency of a pure tone stimulus is a major variable determining its audibility. But how does frequency relate to our discrimination ability? How is our psychological perception of frequency—pitch—related to stimulus frequency and other acoustic variables of a signal? We explore these issues in this section.

In Chapter 7, we explore the phenomenon of masking, learning how the auditory system organizes a stimulus in terms of its frequency components. We see how hearing scientists define and measure masking. We look at the results from important experiments on how various types of auditory signals mask or interfere with the detectability of various pure tones. We relate these findings to the contribution they make to ideas of how frequency information is represented in the peripheral auditory system.

Chapter 8 builds on the masking concept and leads to the development of an important theory regarding the organization of frequency information in the cochlea: the critical band theory. Important experimental evidence concerning the existence of the critical bands, their characteristics, and how they explain our perceptions of complex sounds are dominant in this chapter.

Chapter 9 takes us to issues concerning our discrimination ability for frequency and the important stimulus variables that influence discrimination. We also revisit Weber's law, as it relates to frequency, and compare our relative discrimination ability for intensity versus frequency.

Finally, Chapter 10 explores pitch perception. We see how hearing scientists define the pitch of a stimulus and how estimates of pitch are obtained from human listeners. We examine important studies regarding the role of various stimulus parameters in determining our perceptions of pitch. We take a historical look at theories of pitch perception and their ability to adequately account for our pitch estimates for simple and complex sounds. We end the chapter with an example of a modern-day theory of pitch perception.

The material covered in this section is important. Several of the experiments related to masking are pivotal to the development of major theories for explaining how frequency information is organized and represented in the cochlea and how sounds are represented psychologically. It represents an important era of psychoacoustic investigation that has dominated the field of hearing science for nearly a century.

7

MASKING

■ OVERVIEW

Masking is the effect by which the simultaneous presence of one sound interferes with the detection of another. We all experience masking in everyday listening situations. For instance, when you are speaking with a friend on your cell phone after class, background noise in the listening environment might interfere with your ability to understand what is being said. That is masking: The background noise changes the audibility of the speech signal you're trying to hear. As more students leave the lecture hall and the intensity of the background noise increases, the harder it becomes for you to detect the message. In fact, the intensity of the background noise, relative to the intensity of the conversation you are trying to detect, is a significant acoustic parameter with an enormous influence on your ability to understand speech in everyday listening conditions (Loven and Collins, 1988).

Early studies investigating masking provide insight into how the auditory system processes information regarding *frequency*. By exploring how different kinds of maskers interfere with the audibility of pure tone signals, hearing scientists can infer how the ear processes, represents, and ultimately analyzes information regarding frequency. The results of these early masking experiments, as well as of subsequent studies, have led to the development of an important theory regarding frequency processing in the peripheral auditory system. The **critical band theory**, a cornerstone of psychoacoustic theory, is explored in depth in the next chapter. Masking is the subject of this one.

■ EXPERIMENTAL PARADIGM AND IMPORTANT TERMS

Figure 7-1 shows the fairly straightforward experimental paradigm typically used to demonstrate the masking process. Two auditory stimuli are represented.

1. The **signal** (S) is the stimulus that the listener is trying to detect.

2. The **masker** is the stimulus that may interfere with the detection of the signal.

Usually, the signal is a pure tone, although other types of sounds can be used. Any type of sound can be used as a masker: speech, noise, even other pure tones.

To measure the effect of a masker on a signal, the listener is required to detect the presence of the signal in two different listening conditions.

1. In one condition, the signal is presented *simultaneously* with the masker (represented at the top of Figure 7-1). The experimenter measures the threshold of the signal when presented simultaneously with the masker. This threshold is usually referred to as the **masked threshold.**

2. In the second condition, the signal is presented alone (represented at the bottom of Figure 7-1). The experimenter measures the signal's absolute threshold, which is sometimes referred to as the **threshold in quiet.**

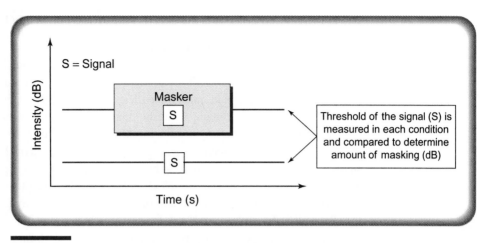

FIGURE 7-1 Typical Experimental Paradigm to Measure the Effect of Simultaneous Masking.

To quantify the effect of the masker on the signal, the experimenter compares the threshold of the signal in quiet to its masked threshold. The difference between these two thresholds is called the **amount of masking** and is expressed in decibels.

Here's an example. Suppose that a scientist is interested in the masking effects of a particular noise on a 1,000-Hz pure tone signal. When the 1,000-Hz signal is presented in quiet, the listener provides a threshold of 22 dB SPL, and the experimenter pairs the 1,000-Hz pure tone with the masker. The researcher again measures the subject's threshold to the signal, this time simultaneously with the masker. The experimenter discovers that the threshold of the 1,000-Hz signal has increased to 57 dB SPL. The difference between the two thresholds (57 dB SPL – 22 dB SPL) is 35 dB. The amount of masking caused by this particular masker at 1,000 Hz is 35 dB.

The magnitude of the amount of masking is directly related to the degree of influence that a masker has on a particular signal. For instance, suppose that the preceding experiment included the masking effects of a second, different noise masker on the 1,000 Hz signal and that the amount of masking measured for the second masker was 20 dB. Here is what we could say about the effectiveness of these two different maskers at 1,000 Hz: Because the magnitude of the amount of masking for the first noise (35 dB) is larger than the amount of masking provided by the second noise (20 dB), the first noise has a greater influence (causes more masking) than the second one. Even though the presence of both maskers interferes with the audibility of the signal, the first masker demonstrates a *greater* interference on the detectability of the 1,000-Hz pure tone than the second. The greater the amount of masking demonstrated in different masking situations, the greater the influence the masker has regarding the audibility of the signal.

SOME CAVEATS REGARDING THE AMOUNT OF MASKING

Suppose a hearing scientist conducts a masking study using the paradigm illustrated in Figure 7-1 and determines that the amount of masking provided by a particular masker for a particular signal is 0 dB. When a masker results in 0 dB of masking, the threshold of the signal in quiet is identical to the threshold of the signal in the presence of the masker. The quiet threshold is the same as the masked threshold. Therefore, we would conclude that the masker has *no effect* on the detectability of the signal. This result may seem surprising, considering that both the masker and the signal are likely audible to the listener, but in this chapter we will explore instances when the presence of a masker doesn't affect the audibility of certain signals. These kinds of experiments provide a lot of information regarding the frequency processing taking place, for both the signal and the masker, in the auditory system.

Can it ever be possible for the amount of masking to be negative? A negative value would imply that the presence of the masker results in a lower (better) threshold to the signal, compared to the quiet condition. Clearly, this could never be the case. The simultaneous presence of a masker with a signal can only work to interfere with signal detection, either impairing audibility or having no effect . As we begin to explore the effects of masker types on the detectability of pure tone signals, keep these caveats in mind.

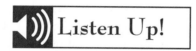 Listen Up!

TECHNICALLY SPEAKING . . .

In this chapter, we are concerned with the effects of a masker when it is presented *simultaneously* with a signal. However, a masker can affect the detectability of a signal if it is presented either a little before or a little after the onset of a signal, a phenomenon referred to as temporal masking or nonsimultaneous masking. Nonsimultaneous masking experiments include conditions where the masker precedes the signal (called forward masking) and conditions where the masker follows the signal (backward masking) (Moore, 2003).

The results from temporal masking studies have significant implications regarding the effect of certain speech sounds on the relative audibility of other speech sounds coming either before or after. This is an area of hearing science that offers important insight into a listener's ability to understand speech in typical listening situations. A relatively new area of psychoacoustic inquiry has captured the attention and enthusiasm of some hearing scientists. Stochastic resonance is an enhancement in the responsiveness of the auditory system when certain noise maskers are presented at appropriate levels (Ries, 2007). While evidence of this beneficial by-product of masking has been repeatedly demonstrated in a handful of studies, the magnitude of the effect is small and the extent to which the auditory system makes use of it remains unclear.

WHEN THE MASKER IS A WIDEBAND NOISE

Hawkins and Stevens (1950) report the results of a simple but elegant study concerning the masking effect of 8 intensity levels of a **wideband noise** masker on 16 pure tone signals, ranging from 100 Hz through 9,000 Hz. You may recall that wideband noise, sometimes called *white noise,* is a complex stimulus that provides equal energy throughout a very broad frequency range. The spectrum of the wideband noise used by Hawkins and Stevens was flat across frequency and ranged in intensity from 20 dB through 90 dB SL. Both the masker and the signal were delivered monaurally, under headphones, to four listeners.

Idealized results from their study are illustrated in Figure 7-2. In the figure, averaged masked thresholds are plotted as a function of signal frequency. The intensity of the wideband noise masker at four levels, in decibel spectrum level, is represented as the parameter of the figure. Sivian and White's (1933) MAP curve is also included for comparison. The salient features from their results include the following:

- *As the intensity of the wideband noise masker increases, the masked pure tone thresholds increase as well,* suggesting that sensitivity to the pure tone signals become poorer. Each time the masker intensity is increased, the intensity

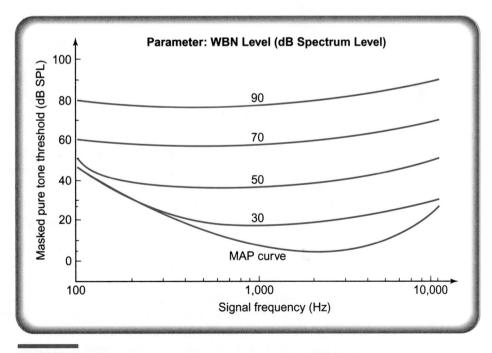

FIGURE 7-2 **Masking Functions of Four Levels of a Wideband Noise Masker on Pure Tone Signals: The threshold of audibility curve is included for reference. (After Hawkins and Stevens, 1950.)**

of the pure tone signals must increase to become detectable again. This is evident for low-, mid-, and high-frequency tones.

- *The masking effects of a wideband noise are not equal across frequency.* Pure tone signals in the mid-frequency range (1,000–3,000 Hz) demonstrate *more masking* compared to low-frequency and high-frequency tones, as demonstrated in the following way. Look at the function corresponding to the lowest-intensity (30 dB) masker in the figure. For very low-frequency pure tone signals (100–300 Hz), the masked thresholds are identical to the threshold of audibility, or the MAP curve; the thresholds of these pure tones in quiet don't change when the masker is present. The amount of masking for these low-frequency signals is 0 dB.

  As signal frequency increases, however, the masked thresholds depart from the threshold of audibility curve. In other words, the amount of masking *increases* as the frequency of the pure tone signals increase from 300 Hz to approximately 5,000 Hz. The biggest departure of the masked threshold function from Sivian and White's MAP function—where the amount of masking is greatest—occurs for pure tone signals between 1,000 and 3,000 Hz.

  As signal frequency increases above 5,000 Hz, the masked threshold function and the MAP function draw closer together, suggesting that the amount of masking provided by this low-level masker decreases for very high-frequency pure tones (5,000–10,000 Hz). Therefore, the presence of a wideband noise masker is most disruptive to the detection of pure tones that correspond to our most sensitive frequency region, the pure tones that correspond to the greatest amount of masking. The presence of a wideband noise masker, although measurable for the higher and lower frequencies, demonstrates a lower amount of masking compared to the middle frequencies.

- *As the presentation level of the wideband noise masker increases, the masked threshold curves become flatter throughout the range of pure tone frequencies investigated.* When the intensity of the masker is low, the masked threshold curve somewhat parallels the threshold of audibility curve. In other words, *masked* pure tone sensitivity is relatively poor in the very low and very high frequencies.

This is not to say that the masker does not affect mid-frequency pure tones. Quite the contrary, as we have just seen, the middle frequencies demonstrate the greatest amount of masking compared to the low and high frequencies. Rather, sensitivity to very low frequency tones and, to a lesser extent, very high frequency tones is poor, whether in the presence of a low-level wideband noise masker or not. As masker intensity increases, however, its effectiveness extends to lower and higher frequencies. Eventually, when the masker level is very intense (90 dB), the influence of the wideband noise masker extends throughout the *entire* audible frequency range, such that sensitivity to pure tones is relatively equal and poor for low-, mid-, and higher-frequency tones.

Essentially, in the presence of a very intense wideband noise masker, our audibility curve flattens out as a function of frequency. We become equally sensitive to the presence of a pure tone, regardless of its frequency. In other words, frequency is no longer an important stimulus variable affecting detection. At lower masker intensities, however, our sensitivity changes with frequency, just as when we listen in quiet; so frequency remains an important acoustic parameter regarding our detection ability. The influence of the signal's frequency becomes less important as the intensity of the wideband noise masker increases.

WHEN THE MASKER IS A PURE TONE

Wegel and Lane (1924) were the first hearing scientists to quantify the masking effects of pure tone maskers on pure tone signals. The results of their experiments were valuable to the development of the critical band theory of frequency analysis, and they reveal important information regarding how the cochlea represents and processes frequency information.

Figure 7-3 illustrates some of the results published by Wegel and Lane. In the figure the effect of a 1,200-Hz pure tone masker on a variety of pure tone signals is illustrated. Three **masking functions** (the amounts of masking as a function of signal frequency) represent the three intensities of the 1,200-Hz masker. Both the masker and the signal were presented monaurally to the listeners by headphones. For each masking function, the amount of masking, in decibels, is plotted as a function of signal frequency. The open circles reflect the actual data points reported by the experimenters, and the solid lines represent a smoothed conceptualization of the masking functions.

The salient points regarding their results in general and Figure 7-3 specifically are as follows:

- *The maximum amount of masking occurs when the signal frequency is very near the frequency of the pure tone masker.* The masker most affects pure tone signals that are slightly lower and slightly higher than 1,200 Hz, the frequency of the pure tone masker. As signal frequency moves farther away from 1,200 Hz, either higher or lower, the amount of masking decreases. When the signal frequency is almost equal to the masker frequency (within a few hertz), the amount of masking appears to decrease significantly. (We'll address these irregularities, or notches, in the masking functions a bit later.) The effectiveness of a pure tone masker appears to be greatest when the signal frequency and the masker frequency are near one another. As the signal frequency moves farther away from the frequency of the pure tone masker, the effectiveness of the masker decreases.

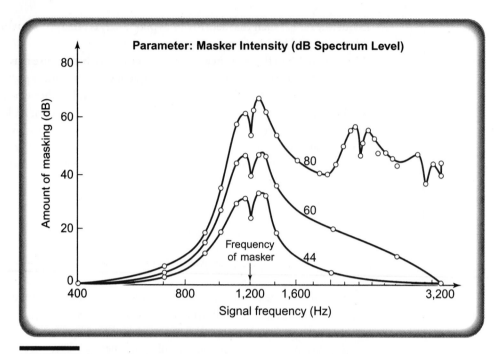

FIGURE 7-3 Masking Functions of Three Levels of a Pure Tone Masker on Pure Tone Signals: Open circles are the actual data points reported by Wegel and Lane (1924). The lines represent an idealized representation of the data. The frequency of the pure tone masker is indicated. (After Wegel and Lane, 1924.)

- *The effectiveness of a pure tone masker is not symmetrical across different signal frequencies.* This is best illustrated by comparing the slopes of the masking functions as masker intensity increases. In Figure 7-3, look at the masking function when the 1,200-Hz masker intensity is low (44 dB SL). When the signal frequency moves away from 1,200 Hz, either higher or lower, the decrease in the amount of masking appears to be somewhat symmetrical. In other words, the slope of the low-frequency side of the masking function is about the same as the slope of the high-frequency side. Now look at the masking functions associated with higher masker intensities: The slopes of the low-frequency sides of the functions compared to those of the high-frequency sides don't appear to be the same. It seems that, as the masker intensity increases from 44 dB SL, through 60 dB SL, to 80 dB SL, the low-frequency sides of the masking pattern becomes steeper, and the high-frequency sides become shallower.

  As the intensity of the masker increases, so does the **asymmetry of masking**, a phenomenon that is referred to as **upward spread of masking** and that highlights the asymmetry of masking by a pure tone. Hearing scientists interpret this phenomenon as suggesting that the effectiveness of a pure tone masker is *greater* for pure tone signals with frequencies higher than the frequency of the masker and *less* for pure tone signals with frequencies lower than the masker frequency. In other words, the masking effect of a pure tone spreads upward in frequency, not downward.

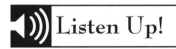 Listen Up!

A PRACTICAL EXERCISE OF UPWARD SPREAD OF MASKING

Here's a practical illustration of upward spread of masking. In Figure 7-3, on the abscissa where signal frequency is plotted, find 800 Hz and 1,600 Hz. These two pure tone signals are both 400 Hz away from the 1,200-Hz masker frequency. One is 400 Hz higher than the frequency of the masker, and the other is 400 Hz lower.

Our aim is to estimate the amount of masking caused by the 1,200-Hz masker for each of these two pure tone signals created as masker intensity is increased. Place a clear ruler vertically at 800 Hz on the *x*-axis, and estimate the amounts of masking by that signal for the three masking functions. You'll need to interpolate the value of the ordinate axis (amount of masking), where each function crosses at 800 Hz. Record your values in the column marked a in Table 7-1; insert the reading for 44 db in the first row, the reading for 60 dB in the second row, and the reading for 80 dB in the bottom row. Repeat the process for the 1,600-Hz signal. Record the values for the amounts of masking at 1,600 Hz for the three masker intensities in the column marked b.

Using the values estimated from Figure 7-3 and presented in Table 7-1, complete Table 7-2. For the first cell in Table 7-2 (under "800 Hz"), place your estimated amount of masking at 800 Hz when the masker intensity is 60 dB SL (row d in Table 7-1) and subtract

TABLE 7-1 **An Exercise in Upward Spread of Masking.**

Masker Intensity(dB SL)	(a) Estimated Amount of Masking at 800 Hz (dB)	(b) Estimated Amount of Masking at 1600 Hz (dB)
(c) 44		
(d) 60		
(e) 80		

TABLE 7-2 Quantifying the Asymmetry of Masking.

Signal Frequency (Hz)		
	800 Hz	1,600 Hz
Change to the amount of masking by increasing masker intensity from 44 to 60 dB SL (d)–(c)		
Change to the amount of masking by increasing masker intensity from 44 to 80 dB SL (e)–(c)		

it from your estimated amount of masking at 800 Hz when the masker intensity is 44 dB SL (row c in Table 7-1). Write this difference in the first upper left cell in Table 7-2. The letters in the first column will help you decide which masker intensities to compare.

Table 7-2 should reflect how the effectiveness of the pure tone masker increases for both signals as the masker intensity increases. If the effectiveness of a masker is directly related to the amount of masking then, as the amount of masking increases with increasing masker intensity, so does the effect of the masker. With each of the signal frequencies represented in Table 7-2, you should notice larger values as you move *down* the rows. Each row represents an increase in the intensity of the masker. The first row corresponds to a 16-dB increase in the masker, and the second row corresponds to a 36-dB increase in masker intensity. Each column should show evidence of a greater amount of masking values as the masker intensity increases. This exercise illustrates the idea that, as a masker increases in intensity, it has an even greater impact on the detectability of a signal. This is evident for signals higher and lower in frequency than that of the masker.

To visualize upward spread of masking, compare the amount of masking values in the first column in Table 7-2 to those in the second column. The changes in the masking values recorded in the second column should be much greater than those in the first column. Because the amount of masking is directly related to the effectiveness of the masker, the 1,200-Hz pure tone masker is *more effective* for the higher-frequency signal (1,600 Hz) than for the lower-frequency signal (800 Hz). This is what hearing scientists mean when they say that the effects of a pure tone masker are asymmetrical. The effectiveness of the masker is much more pronounced for signal frequencies above the masker's frequency than for signal frequencies below the masker's frequency.

- *When the masker and the signal are very close together, the irregularities in the masking functions suggest the perception of* **primary auditory beats**. *When two pure tones that are very similar in frequency are mixed and delivered*

to a subject, the listener perceives the amplitude-modulated signal as beats. Because the subjects in Wegel and Lane's study listened to the pure tone maskers and signals monaurally and simultaneously, they perceived primary auditory beats when the masker and signal were just a few hertz apart. The presence of this additional cue serves to improve the detection of the signal when it is present with the masker. This improvement in detection ability is manifested as a *decrease* in the amount of masking. In other words, the masker was less effective and the signal was more audible when beats were perceived. Once the signal frequency moved far enough away from the frequency of the masker, amplitude modulation was no longer detectable, the additional cue was lost, and the amount of masking increased accordingly. While this idiosyncratic finding in the results reported by Wegel and Lane is not especially pertinent to the masking process, it does point to the remarkable adaptive capabilities of the ear when faced with certain auditory tasks. The ear uses any cue available to improve sensitivity to the presence of a signal.

■ WHEN THE MASKER IS A NARROW BAND OF NOISE

Narrow-band noise, essentially, is wideband noise that is filtered in such a way as to restrict the range of frequencies it covers. We will learn a lot more about filters in the next chapter. For now, understand that narrow-band noise is a complex aperiodic stimulus resulting in a flat continuous spectrum that is restricted to a range of frequencies determined by the experimenter. In terms of its spectral properties, you can think of narrow-band noise as lying between pure tones and wideband noise. Like pure tones, narrow-band noise is limited in its frequency composition. Like wideband noise, it is aperiodic and provides a flat continuous spectrum.

The experimental conditions of Egan and Hake's 1950 study are similar to those of Hawkins and Stevens and Wegel and Lane. Five normal-hearing listeners provided masked thresholds to pure tones in the presence of seven intensities of a narrow-band noise masker. The masker was an extremely limited narrow-band noise centered at 410 Hz and 90 Hz wide. This means that the spectral energy of the noise extended from 365 Hz through 455 Hz. The subjects were presented with seven intensities of the narrow-band noise and of the pure tone signals (there were 29) ranging from 100 Hz to 6,000 Hz. Both the signal and the masker were presented monaurally, under headphones. An illustration of some of Egan and Hake's results appear in Figure 7-4.

The amount of masking, in decibels, is plotted as a function of signal frequency for three intensities of the masker. The open circles represent the data points collected by Egan and Hake, and the solid line represents a smoothed conceptualization of the masking function. Not surprisingly, the important conclusions we can draw from these masking functions is that they include previously discussed characteristics when the masker is a pure tone and when the masker is a wideband noise.

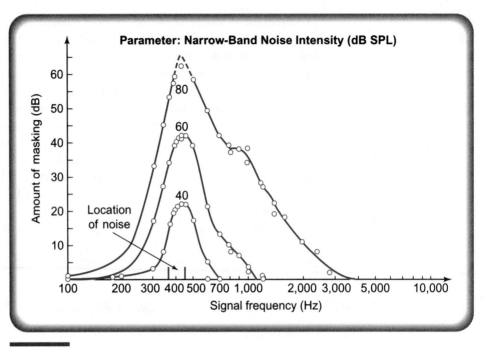

FIGURE 7-4 Masking Functions of Three Levels of a Narrow-Band Noise Masker on Pure
Tone Signals: The closed circles are the actual data points reported by Egan
and Hake (1950). The lines represent an idealized representation of the
data. The location and bandwidth of the narrow-band noise masker are
indicated. (From Jeffress, b1970, after Egan and Hake ,1950.)

- *Like pure tone maskers, the maximum amount of masking with narrow-band noise occurs for pure tone signals whose frequencies fall within the spectral confines of the noise.* Recall that the narrow-band noise used by Egan and Hake contained energy between 365 Hz and 455 Hz. The spectral location of the noise is denoted in Figure 7-4. The pure tone signals whose frequencies fall within the spectrum of the noise band are the ones exhibiting the greatest amount of masking. As the frequency of the pure tone signals move away from the noise band, either up or down, the amount of masking decreases accordingly.

- *Like pure tone maskers, the low-frequency side of the narrow-band noise masking function is steeper than the high-frequency side of the function.* The asymmetry in slope becomes more exaggerated as the masker intensity increases. This implies that the effect of a narrow-band noise masker is asymmetrical and, at high intensity levels, demonstrates upward spread of masking.

- *Like wideband noise maskers, there are no irregularities to the masking function suggesting the presence of primary auditory beats.* Missing from the narrow-band noise masking function is the localized decrease in the amount of masking when the signal frequency is very close to the spectral characteristics of the masker that were evident with pure tone maskers. Remember that amplitude modulation occurs *only* when two *pure tones* of nearly similar frequency are combined. When a pure tone combines with a narrow band of noise, amplitude modulation does not occur, and we do not perceive the presence of beats. There is no additional cue that the ear can use to detect the presence of the signal.

GETTING READY FOR THEORY

Masking, an extremely important concept in psychoacoustic theory, can have a profound influence on our ability to detect sounds, the most basic function of the auditory hierarchy. What we have learned in this chapter about the masking process can be boiled down to two paragraphs:

1. *If the spectral content of the masker is not restricted (think wideband noise), maximum masking occurs within our most sensitive frequency region.* Increasing the intensity of the masker serves to extend its influence to higher- and lower-frequency regions until ultimately masked threshold sensitivity is uniform throughout the entire audible frequency range.

2. *If the spectral content of the masker is restricted (think pure tones and narrow bands of noise), the maximum masking effects occur when the spectral characteristics of the masker and the signal are similar.* In addition, the masking effects of these types of maskers are *asymmetrical* across the frequency range. These maskers tend to have a greater affect on pure tone signals characterized by frequencies higher than the masker's spectral range than on those below it. The asymmetry is most pronounced when the masker intensity is very high.

In the next chapter, we learn how the results of the masking studies reviewed in this chapter, in addition to later studies, are used to help hearing scientists infer how the ear organizes and processes frequency information.

CHAPTER SUMMARY

We have covered several important concepts related to the auditory phenomenon of masking. After reading and studying this chapter, you should be able to do the following:

• Define the process of masking, provide an everyday example of masking in typical listening environments, and explain why an understanding of the masking process is important to hearing scientists.

- Provide an example of a typical experiment used to measure masking, including the sounds presented to the listener, important terms, the listener's task, and how masking is quantified.

- Describe how the effectiveness of a masker is related to the amount of masking.

- Explain why the amount of masking can almost never be a negative value.

- Define wideband noise and identify the three major conclusions regarding the effect of this type of noise on the detection of pure tone signals, as illustrated by the Hawkins and Stevens masking study.

- Define pure tones and identify the three major conclusions regarding the effect of this type of masker on the detection of pure tone signals, as illustrated by Wegel and Lane's masking study.

- Define upward spread of masking and asymmetry of masking, explain how they are related, and describe how these concepts are illustrated by the masking functions reported by Wegel and Lane.

- Explain and describe how the perception of beats was influential to the subjects in Wegel and Lane's masking study.

- Define narrow-band noise and identify the three major conclusions regarding its effect on the detection of pure tone signals, as illustrated by the Egan and Hake masking study.

- Compare and contrast the masking effects of a narrow-band noise to those of a wideband noise masker and to a pure tone masker.

◼ REFERENCES

Egan, J. P., and H. W. Hake. "On the Masking Pattern of Simple Auditory Stimuli." *Journal of the Acoustical Society of America* 35 (1950): 622–630.

Hawkins, J. E., and S. S. Stevens. "The Masking of Pure Tones and Speech by White Noise." *Journal of the Acoustical Society of America* 22 (1950): 6–13.

Jeffress, L. A. "Masking." In *Foundations of Modern Auditory Theory,* Volume I, edited by J. V. Tobias, 87–114. New York: Academic Press, 1970.

Loven, F. C., and M. J. Collins. "Reverberation, Masking, Filtering, and Level Effects on Speech Recognition Performance." *Journal of Speech and Hearing Research* 31 (1988): 681–695.

Moore, B.C.J. *An Introduction to the Psychology of Hearing,* 5th ed. New York: Academic Press, 2003.

Ries, D. T. "The Influence of Noise Type and Level upon Stochastic Resonance in Human Audition." *Hearing Research* 228 (2007): 136–143.

Sivian, L. J., and S. D. White. "On Minimum Audible Sound Fields." *Journal of the Acoustical Society of America* 4 (1933): 288–321.

Wegel, R. L., and C. E. Lane. "The Auditory Masking of One Pure Tone by Another and Its Probable Relation to the Dynamics of the Inner Ear." *Physics Review* 23 (1924): 266–285.

8

FREQUENCY SELECTIVITY AND THE CRITICAL BAND

OVERVIEW

Clearly, the effectiveness of a masker very much depends on the relationship between spectral content of the masker and the signal. For maskers characterized by spectral limiting (pure tones and narrow bands of noise), maximum masking occurs when the frequency of the pure tone signal closely matches the spectral components of the masker. When the spectral characteristics of the masker and the signal don't match very well, the effectiveness of the masker is restricted; sometimes the masker is rendered completely ineffective in altering pure tone sensitivity from quiet conditions. This behavior, as observed by hearing scientists, suggests that the ear treats sounds differently based on their spectral content. In other words, the ear is said to be frequency selective in terms of how it organizes, represents, and analyzes acoustic events reaching the cochlea.

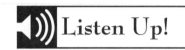

TONOTOPIC ORGANIZATION OF THE PERIPHERAL AUDITORY SYSTEM

The ear organizes, represents, and analyzes sounds differently based on the frequency components making up the stimulus. This is the basic premise of **tonotopic organization**, which is the theory that tones close to each other in terms of frequency are represented in topologically neighboring places at the level of the basilar membrane and beyond. (Literally, "tonotopic" means the "place of tones.") Evidence of tonotopic organization is seen in the traveling wave response of the basilar membrane. Recall that high-frequency sounds typically show maximum excitation of the basilar membrane at the base of the cochlea, and low-frequency sounds demonstrate maximum excitation of the membrane corresponding to the apex.

Research over the last half century has supported this theory. Von Bekesy (1960) determined that the unique physical characteristics of the basilar membrane, namely the stiffness gradient, give rise to its topologic response. In addition, strong evidence of tonotopic organization is seen in the neurological response of the first-order auditory neurons innervating the hair cells of the basilar membrane. Kiang and colleagues (1965) were among the first scientists to show the frequency response patterns of single-fiber auditory neurons. These nerve fibers, innervating the individual hair cells within the cochlea, are very frequency selective; that is, if a single neuron is going to respond (fire) to an auditory stimulus, it does so only for a relatively limited range of stimulus frequencies. Again, the single auditory nerve fibers that are the most responsive to high-frequency sounds are located near the base of the cochlea; fibers that are the most responsive to low-frequency sounds arise from the apex. There is also considerable evidence of tonotopic organization at higher levels of the auditory system (Pickles, 1988). Although the scientific evidence of tonotopic organization in the central pathways of the ear was not reported until the latter half of the twentieth century, evidence of this kind of frequency-selective organization involving the mechanical properties of the cochlea and the first-order auditory neurons came a few decades sooner.

Hearing scientists had long been familiar with an electronic device that behaves similarly to the ear in it changes the characteristics of incoming signals based on spectral content. The device, called a filter, has been around for a long time; so it was natural for early hearing scientists to think of the ear as acting like a filter. The question was what primary characteristics of an internal auditory filter can explain the masking behaviors that we see empirically? The **critical band theory** addresses this question. This theory explains the frequency selectivity of the cochlea as a filter—or, more accurately, as a series of filters—at the anatomical level of the basilar membrane.

In this chapter we explore the simple beginnings of the critical band theory and how early hearing scientists were able to define the basic characteristics of the critical bands. We see how this theory explains the behaviors of maskers, as well as our perceptions of other complex sounds. We begin with a brief overview of filters and their important characteristics.

FILTERS

Electronic filters have been in existence for some time. Their purpose is to remove unwanted energy from a signal and allow for the transmission of the desired energy, based on the frequency components of the signal entering the filter. A **filter** is a frequency-selective attenuating device. Depending on the characteristics of the filter, usually determined by its purpose, it allows some spectral energy to pass (i.e., does not reduce original amplitude) and attenuates some spectral energy (i.e., reduces the original amplitude). Whether energy is allowed to pass depends on the signal's frequency components and on the filter's characteristics.

Depending on its purpose, the frequency-selective attenuating properties of a filter can vary. We review three basic kinds of filters and define their important characteristics:

1. High-pass filters
2. Low-pass filters
3. Band-pass filters

HIGH-PASS FILTERS

In some engineering applications, the low-frequency components of a signal have to be removed. For this purpose, a **high-pass filter** can be employed. We all have encountered a high-pass filter when using any sort of radio, CD player,

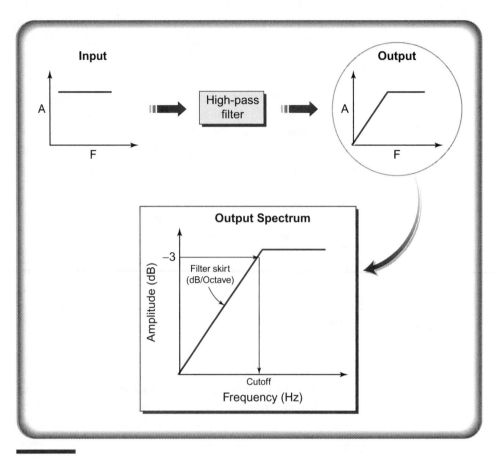

FIGURE 8-1   The Effects of High-Pass Filtering: When a flat input spectrum is passed
             through a high-pass filter, the filtered output spectrum is enlarged.

or MP3 player. Most of these devices have some degree of control over the
amount of bass (or low frequency) you hear. By adjusting the bass control, you
are probably employing a high-pass filter, which attenuates the low-frequency
components of a signal and allows the high-frequency components to pass
unattenuated.

The effects of a high-pass filter and its important characteristics are illustrated
in Figure 8-1, which shows the effect of a high-pass filter on a signal with a
flat spectrum. The spectrum of the signal entering the filter, the **input signal**,
is characterized by equal energy across a broad frequency range. After passing
through the high-pass filter, the spectrum of the input signal has changed. We
see that the low frequencies have been attenuated and that the high frequencies
have been allowed to pass without any change. The new spectrum is the **output
signal**, or the signal coming out of the filter.

Important Characteristics of High-Pass Filters

Figure 8-1 illustrates the output spectrum of a high-pass filter and the important landmarks of this spectrum. As denoted in the figure, the important characteristics of this filter are its

- Cutoff frequency
- Filter skirt (rejection rate)

The filter's **cutoff frequency** is the critical frequency at which spectral energy will either be attenuated or allowed to pass through unchanged. You can think of this as the critical frequency at which the filter becomes active. The cutoff frequency is determined by finding where a 3-dB decrease in output signal amplitude corresponds with the filter's spectrum and interpolating the frequency where this occurs, as illustrated in Figure 8-1. A 3-dB reduction in amplitude (usually expressed in power) represents an intensity reduction of half the original intensity of the signal. Hearing scientists usually refer to this as the **3-dB down point**. The important point is that, for a high-pass filter, the cutoff frequency tells us where the attenuating characteristics of the filter kick in.

- The frequency components of the input signal lower than the cutoff frequency are attenuated.
- The frequency components of the input signal higher than the filter's cutoff frequency are not attenuated, and these frequencies pass at full amplitude.

The **filter skirt** of a high-pass filter represents the region of the filter's spectrum to the *left* of the cutoff frequency, that is, the frequency region that corresponds to frequency-selective attenuation. To understand a filter skirt, we must define the term rejection rate. The **rejection rate** is a quantitative measure of the slope of the filter skirt, expressed as decibels per octave (dB/octave). An octave is the interval between one pure tone and another with half or double its frequency. The larger the rejection rate's magnitude, the steeper the slope of the filter skirt. For example, a high-pass filter with a rejection rate of 32 dB/octave has a much steeper filter skirt than a high-pass filter with a rejection rage of 8 dB/octave. The rejection rate magnitude of a high-pass filter's skirt allows us to infer how much attenuation will take place in the frequency components of an input signal whose frequencies lie *below* the cutoff level.

- If the rejection rate is a large value, then components of the input signal much lower than the cutoff frequency of the filter experience a lot of attenuation.
- If the rejection rate is a small value, then frequencies lower than the cutoff frequency of the filter, although attenuated compared to its input level, may still pass through with some degree of amplitude.

LOW-PASS FILTERS

A **low-pass filter**, as you might guess, allows low frequencies of the input signal to pass unattenuated, while restricting the passage of high-frequency energy. This kind of filter might be employed if the intent is to remove high-frequency information from the input signal. For example, a treble control on your CD player enables you to reduce the high frequencies (i.e., decrease the treble); the treble control is probably a low-pass filter.

Figure 8-2 illustrates the effects of a low-pass filter on a flat spectrum input signal. When this type of input signal is passed through a low-pass filter, the output spectrum shows low-frequency components passing unattenuated, while the high-frequency components are restricted.

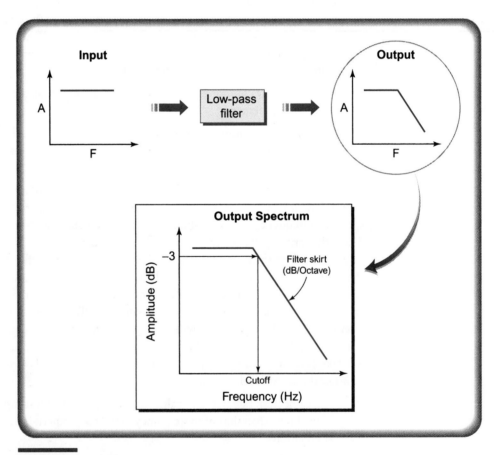

FIGURE 8-2 The Effects of Low-Pass Filtering: When a flat input spectrum is passed through a low-pass filter, the filtered output spectrum is enlarged.

Important Characteristics of Low-Pass Filters

As with high-pass filters, low-pass filters share similar important characteristics, which are also identified in Figure 8-2.

The cutoff frequency of a low-pass filter represents the critical frequency at which the effects of the filter kick in. It is found where the 3-dB down point on the ordinate intersects the filter spectrum. For low-pass filters, frequencies components of the input signal *lower* than the cutoff frequency are allowed to pass unattenuated. Input signal frequency components higher than the cutoff frequency are restricted.

Low-pass filters are also characterized by a filter skirt, located to the *right* of the cutoff frequency on the output spectrum. This is the frequency region where the filter is attenuating the higher-frequency components of the input signal. Again, the magnitude of the degree of filtering is taken as the slope of the filter skirt (dB/octave) and referred to as the rejection rate. The larger the rejection rate, the more attenuation we see for frequencies higher than the filter's cutoff frequency.

BAND-PASS FILTERS

Suppose an engineer passes a flat spectrum input signal first through a high-pass filter and then through a low-pass filter. Figure 8-3 illustrates what the output spectrum of the new signal would look like. After passing through the high-pass filter, a spectrum similar to the output spectrum shown in Figure 8-1 results. When that output spectrum is passed through a low-pass filter (like the one shown in Figure 8-2), the final outcome is an output spectrum that shows evidence of the combined effect of the two filters: what we call a **band-pass filter**. As the name implies, a band-pass filter attenuates input signal frequency components at the high *and* low frequencies. The result is that only a band of frequencies is allowed to pass unattenuated. Input frequencies above and below the pass band are attenuated. Band-pass filters are made by passing an input signal through high- and low-pass filters in succession.

Important Characteristics of Band-Pass Filters

Figure 8-4 illustrates a typical output spectrum from a band-pass filter.

- *Center frequency:* By definition, band-pass filters allow a relatively restricted range of input frequencies to pass through unattenuated. The single frequency lying in the exact center of this band is referred to as the **center frequency**. You can think of this frequency as the pivot frequency on which the filter is centered or the frequency over which the filter is directly centered.

- *Lower cutoff frequency:* The **lower cutoff frequency** is the lower frequency limit of the pass band. Input signal component frequencies below the lower cutoff frequency are attenuated. The lower cutoff frequency is determined

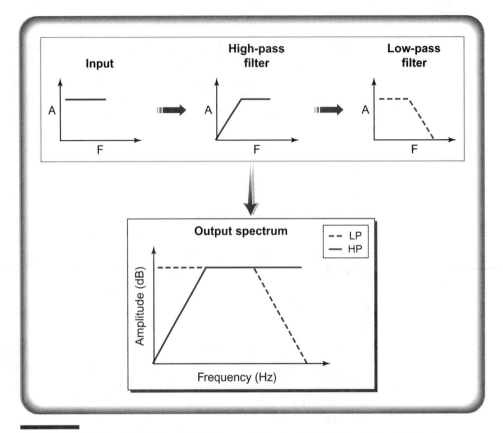

FIGURE 8-3 A Band-Pass Filter: A band-pass filter is made by running a flat input
spectrum through high- and low-pass filters in series. The resulting output
spectrum is enlarged.

by the cutoff frequency of the high-pass filter in the filter series, and it is
measured in the same manner. The frequency corresponding to the 3-dB
down point on the left side of the band-pass spectrum is interpolated
from the output spectrum; this is the lower cutoff frequency of the
band-pass filter.

- *Higher cutoff frequency:* The **higher cutoff frequency** is the upper frequency
  limit of the pass band, and it is determined by the cutoff frequency of the
  low-pass filter of the filter series. Input signal frequencies higher than the
  higher cutoff frequency are attenuated; input frequencies below it are not.

- *Bandwidth:* A very important characteristic, the **bandwidth** of a band-pass
  filter is essentially the width of the frequency band that is allowed to pass
  without reduction in amplitude. The bandwidth is calculated by taking the
  difference between the higher cutoff frequency and lower cutoff frequency

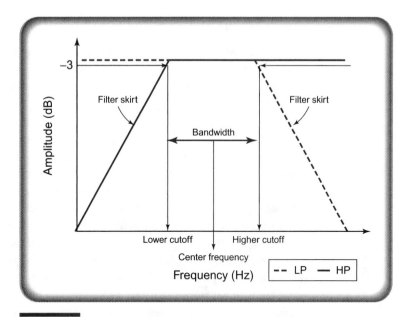

FIGURE 8-4 Important Characteristics of a Band-Pass Filter.

of the band-pass output spectrum, and it is measured in hertz. If the bandwidth is relatively narrow, the filter is described as being highly tuned—in a sense, being very selective, or choosy, about the frequency components allowed to pass through the filter unchanged. On the other hand, if the bandwidth is relatively wide, then the filter is said to be broadly tuned—less selective in terms of the frequency range allowed to pass. More frequency components of the input signal are allowed to pass without change. The magnitude of the bandwidth quantifies the degree of tuning, or selectivity, of the band-pass filter. The center frequency of the filter should fall in the exact center of the bandwidth. In other words, one-half of the bandwidth of the filter lies above the center frequency, and one-half lies below it.

- *Filter skirt:* The filter skirts of a band-pass filter, as in high- and low-pass filters, indicate the frequency regions where attenuation takes place; a band-pass filter has *two* filter skirts. One skirt, on the lower-frequency side of the output spectrum, is determined by the high-pass skirt of the filter series. The filter skirt on the higher-frequency side is determined by the characteristics of the low-pass skirt. Figure 8-4 illustrates symmetrical filter skirts. The rejection rates of both the high- and low-pass filters are the same. This is not always the case, depending on the purpose of the band-pass filter. Sometimes the rejection rates of the low- and high-frequency sides of a band-pass filter are different.

■ EARLY WORK ON THE CRITICAL BAND THEORY

In 1940, Harvey Fletcher published a paper reporting the results of experimental work he had conducted at Bell Laboratories. In this historic paper, Fletcher (1940) laid the groundwork for the basis of the critical band theory and its inference regarding the frequency selectivity of the cochlea. Fletcher presented a model of auditory patterns produced at the basilar membrane in response to various pure tones at numerous intensities. He built his model of auditory patterns on the assumption that the cochlea processes frequency information in discrete "chunks" along the length of the basilar membrane. He hypothesized that each ½-mm length along the basilar membrane, in essence, represented a separate and discrete internal auditory band-pass filter. His dilemma was that the characteristics of these hypothetical filters would have to change from the base to the apex of the basilar membrane to take into account the empirical observations by Wegel and Lane (1924) and other data available at the time describing normal human frequency discrimination. (We discuss frequency discrimination ability in the next chapter.) The major sticking point for Fletcher from the Wegel and Lane pure tone masking data was that the masking functions of low-frequency pure tone maskers were *narrower* than those from high-frequency pure tone maskers. In other words, the bandwidth of signal frequencies significantly affected by a pure tone maker was greater (wider) when the masker frequency was relatively high, compared to lower masker frequencies. This was especially true for pure tone maskers above 1,000 Hz.

Fletcher proposed the following theory regarding frequency processing in the cochlea: The basilar membrane can be thought of as a number of band-pass filters arranged serially according to center frequency. As we move down the length of the membrane, from base to apex, the center frequency of the band-pass filters decreases progressively, from high frequencies to low. Each ½ mm traveled represents a move to the next adjacent band-pass filter, or **critical band**. To account for the masking data collected by Wegel and Lane, Fletcher hypothesized that the bandwidths of these critical bands become *wider* as the center frequency *increases*. In other words, the **critical bandwidth** of these internal filters must be relatively wide at the base of the cochlea, the place where high frequencies demonstrate maximum excitation of the traveling wave, and become progressively narrower toward the apex of the cochlea, the place where low frequencies demonstrate maximum excitation of the traveling wave. Fletcher devised a landmark masking study to test his hypothesis.

FLETCHER'S LOGIC

There's an important caveat to Fletcher's hypothesis. He assumed that, in the case of a pure tone signal just masked by the presence of a noise, the energy of the pure tone signal and the energy of the noise within a single critical band must be equal. Figure 8-5 illustrates his logic. If we present the ear with a 1,000-Hz pure tone, Fletcher hypothesized that the energy of this signal would be represented in the critical band filter centered at 1,000 Hz. Once the energy of the tone reaches some critical power level, within this one critical band, the tone becomes audible. In the top panel of Figure 8-5, the pure tone has reached critical power within this one critical band and becomes detectable.

The addition of the simultaneous presence of a wideband noise masker at a low-intensity level is depicted in the second panel of Figure 8-5. The noise spectrum exists across the entire audible range, adding some noise to all the critical bands throughout the length of the cochlea, including the critical band centered on the pure tone signal. Fletcher would predict that, since the noise energy within the critical band centered around 1,000 Hz has increased, the energy of the 1,000-Hz signal needs to increase proportionately to keep the tone audible. According to Fletcher, the energy of the noise and the energy of the pure tone, within this one critical band, must remain at least equal for detection of the pure tone to occur.

Let's increase the intensity of the wideband noise such that it reaches the top of the critical band centered at 1,000 Hz. To keep the pure tone energy equal to the energy of noise in the band, the intensity of the tone needs to increase, compared to when the noise was at a lower intensity level, as illustrated in the third panel of Figure 8-5. Other critical bands fill as well, but they aren't involved in the detection of this particular pure tone. This is just the behavior we observe when looking at the effects of a wideband noise masker on pure tones. You may want to look again at Figure 7-2, where Hawkins and Stevens' (1950) masking functions for various levels of a wideband noise masker are illustrated. Clearly, once a pure tone signal's sensitivity is affected by the presence of the masker, further increases to the masker's intensity bring about a proportional increase in the masked threshold of the signal. Fletcher appears to be on the right track.

The final panel of Figure 8-5 highlights the important contribution of Fletcher's critical band theory. Here, the intensity of the wideband noise is increased beyond what is evident in the previous panel. Because the noise energy and the tone are equal within the critical band centered at 1,000 Hz in the previous panel, further increases in the intensity of the noise make no change in the relationship between the signal and the noise *within this one critical band*. Fletcher would argue that the masked threshold of the pure tone, between panels c and d of Figure 8-5, would remain the same. The intensity of the noise in panel c fills the critical band; so increasing the intensity of the masker, doesn't change anything as far as that one critical band is concerned. In fact, it's affecting the noise level in only adjacent critical bands, not *the* critical band responsible for providing information about the 1,000-Hz signal. The critical band theory suggests that this is the only critical band, the only region of the basilar membrane that the ear is looking at to make decisions about the audibility of the 1,000-Hz pure tone. Once the critical band responsible for the detection of a single pure tone is full, further increases in masker energy won't bring about any change in pure tone threshold. However, if the

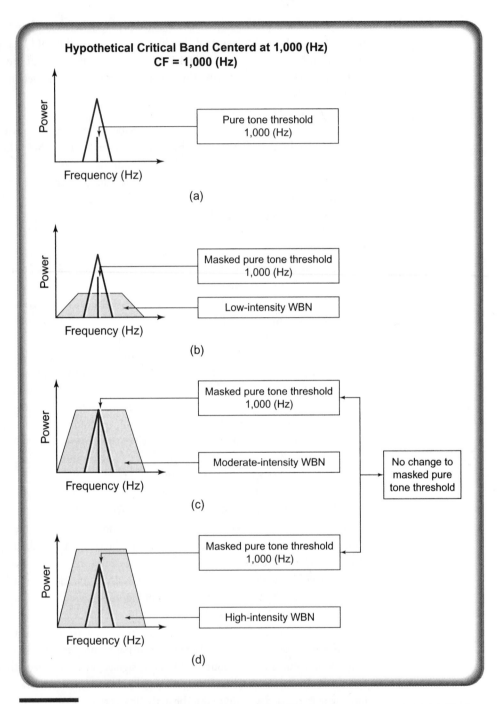

FIGURE 8-5 Fletcher's (1940) Logic Regarding the Audibility of Pure Tones in the Critical
Bands: (a) The audible 1,000-Hz pure tone is centered on the critical band with
a 1,000-Hz center frequency. Fletcher (1940) would maintain that the overall

(Continues)

noise energy within that single critical band is reduced, masked pure tone threshold decreases proportionately.

Fletcher's Masking Study

To confirm his logic concerning the existence and characteristics of critical bands, Fletcher performed the following masking study. Masked pure tone thresholds were obtained from listeners for a variety of pure tone signals in the simultaneous presence of a wideband noise masker. Figure 8-6 provides a schematic of the spectra of the masker and of the signals presented to the listeners. The important variable of his study is the change he made to the bandwidth of the wideband noise. Fletcher systematically removed the upper and lower ends of the wideband noise, all the while checking the masked threshold of the pure tone in the center of the noise band. Essentially, the wideband noise was changed to a narrow-band noise masker, always centered on the frequency of the pure tone signal. The masker was eventually narrowed to a 20-Hz bandwidth, all the while keeping track of the masked threshold for the pure tone. Fletcher repeated this process for a variety of pure tone signals ranging in frequency from 125 Hz to 8,000 Hz.

His results are shown in Figure 8-7, which plots a masked pure tone threshold as a function of the noise bandwidth. The parameter of the graph is the frequency of the pure tone signals. The figure shows that the results support his hypothesis that the bandwidths of the critical bands are wider for critical bands centered at higher frequencies, compared to lower center frequency critical bands. However, you may need a little help with interpreting the presentation of his results. To help you, in the figure, locate the function corresponding to the 2,000-Hz pure tone signal, which corresponds to the straight line determined from the open square data points. Starting from the *right side* of the abscissa (noise bandwidth), follow the course of the masked pure tone threshold as the bandwidth of the noise *decreases*. In other words, follow the 2,000-Hz function from the right side of the figure to the

---

FIGURE 8-5 **(Continued)** power of the pure tone must exceed a minimum level within the critical band audible. (b) An audible 1,000-Hz pure tone in the presence of a low-level wideband noise masker. Notice that the intensity of the pure tone must increase to keep the tone audible. Fletcher would hypothesize that the overall power of the pure tone must exceed the power of the masker in the critical band to be detected. (c) An audible 1,000-Hz pure tone in the presence of a moderate-level wideband noise masker. The intensity of the pure tone must increase again to keep the tone audible, and the masker and the tone are at the top of the critical band centered on 1,000 Hz. (d) An audible 1,000-Hz pure tone in the presence of a high-intensity wideband noise masker. Fletcher would argue that the masked pure tone threshold will not change from the previous panel because the critical band is full. Increasing the level of the masker only serves to increase the noise power in adjacent critical bands, not the critical band responsible for detection of the 1,000-Hz tone. Therefore, the masked threshold will not increase from the conditions illustrated in (c).

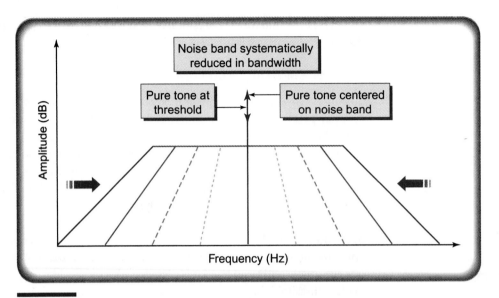

FIGURE 8-6 Fletcher's (1940) Masking Study: Subjects were presented with a single pure tone signal embedded in a wideband noise (dark line spectrum). Masked pure tone threshold was obtained. The bandwidth of the wideband noise spectrum was systematically reduced, equally on the high- and low-frequency sides, all the while keeping the masked pure tone at threshold. The subsequent noise spectrum throughout the course of the study is represented by the various dotted lines. Notice that the pure tone is always in the center of the noise band. (From Small, 1973, after Fletcher, 1940.)

left. The bandwidth of the noise masker decreases, and the masked threshold for the 2,000-Hz signal remains constant. In fact, masked pure tone threshold remains constant through masker bandwidths from 20,000 Hz all the way down to 100 Hz. However, once the bandwidth of the noise reaches 100 Hz, the masked threshold of the 2,000-Hz pure tone signal decreases linearly as the noise bandwidth is reduced further. Look at the change in masked pure tone thresholds to the other pure tone signals representing the parameter of the graph: They all do the same thing. When the bandwidth of the noise is wide, masked pure tone threshold is high. As the bandwidth of the noise decreases, always centered on the frequency of the pure tone signal, masked threshold remains constant *until* reaching a critical bandwidth of the masker. At this point, further reduction in the bandwidth of the noise brings about a proportional decrease in the masked threshold of the signal.

Fletcher's hypothesis regarding the characteristics of the critical bands with center frequencies is supported. Figure 8-7 shows the bandwidth of the masker at which the masked threshold of the pure tone signal changes from a constant intensity to decreasing intensity at a discrete frequency. The actual bandwidth of the masker where this change in threshold occurs, however, varies with the frequency of the signal. Higher pure tone signals intersect the knee of the function at larger (wider) bandwidths, compared to lower signal frequencies.

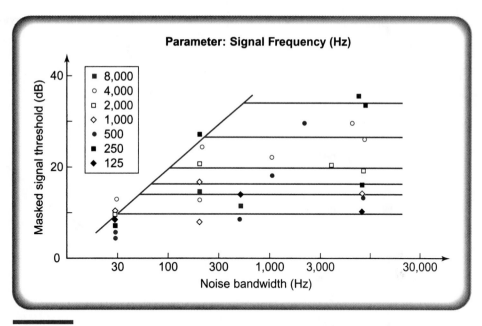

FIGURE 8-7 **Fletcher's (1940) Masking Functions:** Masked pure tone thresholds are plotted as a function of masker noise bandwith. The parameter is the frequency of the pure tone signal. Regardless of signal frequency, masked threshold remains constant as the noise bandwidth decreases, until a critical bandwith is reached, then it decreases, and masked threshold decreases linearly. The critical bandwidth is dependent on the frequency of the pure tone signal. Higher-frequency pure tone signals are affected by wider bandwidths of the noise, compared to lower-frequency pure tone signals. Fletcher (1940) argued that the bandwidth of the noise corresponding to the change in masked pure tone threshold estimates the bandwidth of the critical band at the center frequency of the signal. (After Fletcher, 1940.)

FLETCHER'S LEGACY

Fletcher's original work regarding the critical bands has been replicated numerous times over the years, using a variety of psychophysical methods other than simultaneous masking. A compilation of several investigations reporting the bandwidths of the critical bands as a function of center (signal) frequency is illustrated in Figure 8-8 (Greenwood, 1961; Hawkins and Stevens, 1950; Scharf, 1961; Zwicker, Flottorp, and Stevens, 1957). The data points refer to the actual bandwidth values obtained by the investigators cited. The function represents a smoothed line of the collective results. Although the debate continues among hearing scientists regarding the exact widths of the critical bands and their theoretical interpretation as an auditory filter (Scharf, 1970), the basic conclusions reported by Fletcher are still upheld today.

Figure 8-8 summarizes the important characteristics of the critical bands very well. Namely, the bandwidth of the critical bands are roughly constant, about

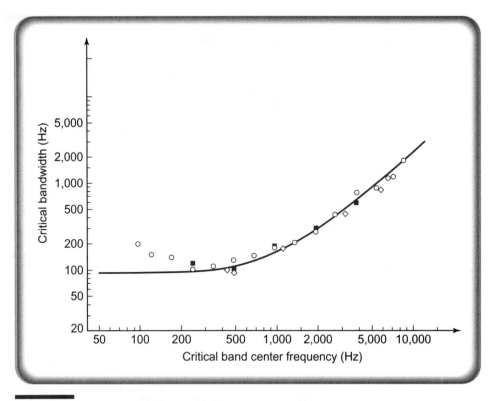

FIGURE 8-8 Average Critical Bandwidth as a Function of the Center Frequency of the Band: Data from a number of different studies measuring critical bandwidth as a function of center frequency are represented, with a variety of different psychophysical procedures employed. (From Scharf, 1970.)

100 Hz wide, for center frequencies from 50 Hz through 500 Hz. As the center frequency of the critical band increases (as we move closer to the base of the cochlea), the bandwidth increases steadily, such that by the time we reach 10,000 Hz, the bandwidth is estimated to be about 2,000 Hz wide. What does this suggest regarding the *tuning* of the critical band mechanism at the level of the basilar membrane? Recall two facts: (1) The magnitude of a filter's bandwidth is a numerical representation of the degree of tuning, or frequency selectivity; (2) the narrower the bandwidth, the more selective, or choosy, the filter is in allowing frequency components to pass through unattenuated. The wider the bandwidth, the less selective the filter is assumed to be. Using this logic, the critical bands at the apex of the cochlea (the low-frequency end) demonstrate *more tuning* compared to critical bands at the base of the cochlea (the high-frequency end). Moreover, as we travel from the apex of the cochlea to the base, critical bandwidth increases steadily, suggesting that the degree of tuning *decreases* and that frequency selectivity becomes

poorer. (In the next chapter, we see that this has important implications regarding our frequency discrimination ability, as a function of signal frequency.)

Further Evidence of the Critical Band: Loudness Summation

We have other perceptions of complex sounds that appear to corroborate the existence of the critical bands. Suppose an experimenter presented a listener with an audible narrow band of noise, centered on 1,000 Hz with a bandwidth of 50 Hz, and the listener provides a loudness estimate of this noise using a loudness balance procedure (see Chapter 5). The experimenter systematically increases the bandwidth of the noise band, keeping the noise centered on 1,000 Hz and keeping the overall energy of the noise constant. With each increase in the bandwidth, the listener provides a loudness estimate of the noise. Does the loudness of the narrow band noise change as the bandwidth of the noise is increased—or does it stay constant?

The results of such a study, presented in Figure 8-9, come from a study by Feldtkeller and Zwicker (1956). Plotted are loudness estimates, in phons, of narrow

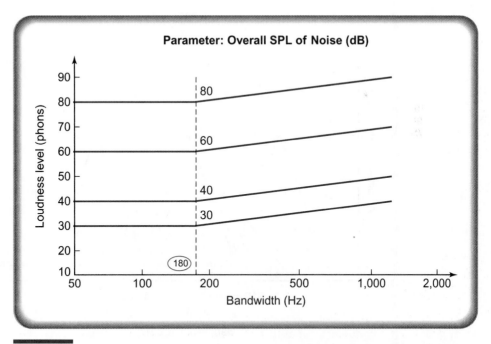

FIGURE 8-9 Empirical Evidence of Loudness Summation: Loudness estimates of various levels of noise are plotted as a function of the bandwidth of the noise, centered on 1,000 Hz. The loudness estimate of the noise remains constant, with bandwidth, until the bandwidth exceeds a critical value (180 Hz), then loudness increases. The overall intensity of the noise doesn't seem to affect the trend. (From Scharf, 1970, after Feldtkeller and Zwicker, 1956.)

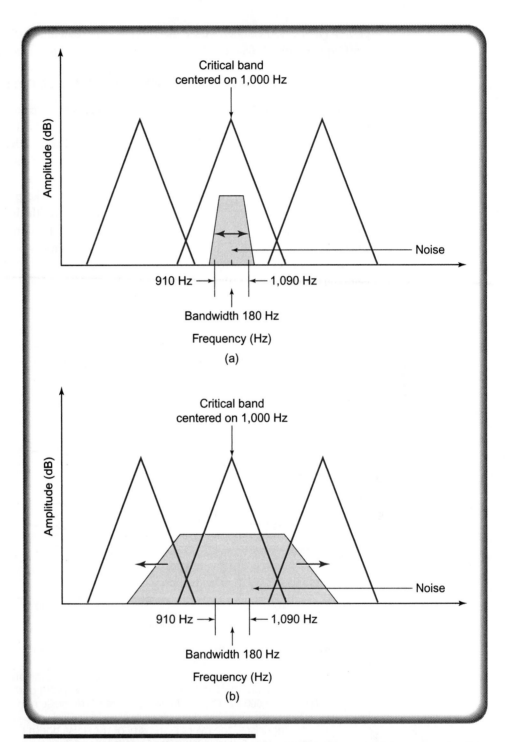

FIGURE 8-10 Loudness Summation: (a) The critical band with center frequency of 1,000
Hz, with the two adjacent critical bands higher and lower in center

(Continues)

bands of noise as a function of noise bandwidth. The parameter of the graph is the overall sound pressure level of the noise, from 30 dB through 80 dB. These results suggest that the loudness of the noise band remains constant until the bandwidth exceeds 180 Hz (illustrated in the figure by the dashed vertical line). As the bandwidth is increased, the loudness of the noise increases, apparently regardless of the overall intensity of the noise. The critical bandwidth at which loudness begins to increase appears to remain at 180 Hz.

This auditory phenomenon—increasing loudness of a noise with increasing bandwidth once a critical bandwidth is achieved—is called **loudness summation**. First reported by Zwicker, Flottorp, and Stevens in 1957 and replicated many times since then, loudness summation is well explained by the existence of the critical bands. The results shown in Figure 8-9 (loudness summation for noise bands centered on 1,000 Hz) suggest that, as long as the noise bandwidth remains narrower than 180 Hz, the loudness of the noise remains constant. However, once the bandwidth of the noise exceeds 180 Hz, any further increase in noise bandwidth beyond this critical value brings about a corresponding increase in loudness. In other words, beyond the critical bandwidth of 180 Hz (centered on 1,000 Hz), the loudness of the noise appears to summate (add) as the bandwidth increases.

The explanation of loudness summation, using critical bands, is illustrated in Figure 8-10. In this figure, three adjacent critical bands are represented: the critical band with center frequency at 1,000 Hz and the two adjacent critical bands to the right (higher frequency) and the left (lower frequency). Experimental evidence of the critical band centered on 1,000 Hz suggests that it is about 180 Hz wide (see Figure 8-8); the hypothetical upper and lower cutoff frequencies of the 1,000 Hz critical band are included in Figure 8-10. When the loudness of the noise remains constant with bandwidths ranging from 50 Hz to 180 Hz, the noise is contained within the critical band centered on 1,000 Hz. As the bandwidth is adjusted wider or narrower within this critical band, loudness remains constant, as long *as the overall energy of the noise remains the same* (top panel of the figure). In other words, as long as nothing is changing within this *one* critical band, perception does not change. However, once the bandwidth of the noise exceeds 180 Hz (the lower panel in the figure), the noise spills into adjacent critical bands. When this occurs, we perceive an increase in the loudness of the noise. It's thought that

FIGURE 8-10 *(Continued)* frequency and a narrow band of noise within the limits of the center critical bands. As the noise bandwidth increases and decreases, the loudness of the noise does not change as long as the noise remains within the bandwidth of the center critical band. Note the upper and lower cutoff frequencies of the critical band centered on 1,000 Hz. (b) With the presence of a noise whose bandwidth exceeds the critical bandwidth centered on 1,000 Hz, the noise energy has spilled into the adjacent critical band. The loudness of the noise increases in this condition, suggesting that noise energy in adjacent critical bands summate, or add, to increase the perceived loudness of the noise. The overall power of the noise in either panel is the same.

the ear summates, or adds, the energy contained within adjacent critical bands. As a result, the overall energy representation of the noise increases and is perceived as an increase in loudness.

Further Evidence of the Critical Band: Threshold, Tonal Separation, and Component Bandwidth of Complex Periodic Signals

We have seen from Fletcher's masking study that masking energy outside a single critical band does not contribute to the masking of a signal within that band. Further evidence suggests that it also may not contribute to the detection of a complex, periodic sound. In 1954, Gassler measured detection thresholds of multiple pure tone complexes in normal-hearing listeners. The complex signal was composed of 1 through 40 pure tones evenly spaced 10 Hz or 20 Hz apart and centered on 1,000 Hz. Gassler (1954) was interested to learn if the number of pure tone components present in the signal had any bearing on the overall threshold of the complex. He found that, as long as the frequency spacing among all the components of the complex stayed within a 200-Hz bandwidth, detection threshold remained constant. In other words, adding more pure tone components to the complex periodic signal resulted in no change to the overall sound pressure level of the signal necessary for detection.

In Figure 8-8, the bandwidth of the critical band centered on 1,000 Hz is about 200 Hz wide. Once the overall frequency spacing of the pure tone components exceed a 200-Hz bandwidth, however, absolute threshold to the signal increases. In addition, as more pure tones are systematically added to the complex, detection threshold of the complex increase further.

Gassler interpreted these results as suggesting that signal energy within adjacent critical bands does not summate to aid the listener in detecting the signal. In other words, as long as the multiple pure tone components of the signal fall within the bandwidth of a single critical band, their respective energies add, or summate. And, as long as the overall power of the signal remains constant as additional components are added to the complex, threshold to the complex remains constant. However, once the complex includes pure tone components exceeding the bandwidth of the critical band, the additional power or energy of these pure tones does not add with the others; so threshold increases, suggesting that more power is needed within the critical band at 1,000 Hz to keep the signal audible. This suggests that only the pure tones falling within the one critical band under observation by the ear are responsible for detection. As additional components are added beyond the critical band, the intensity of the components within the critical band must be increased to keep them audible.

Since Gassler's report, a number of investigators have tried to replicate these findings. Subsequent studies suggest that audibility changes as the frequency spacing or number of the pure tone components exceed the bandwidth of the critical band surrounding the signal frequency. There is considerable disagreement, however,

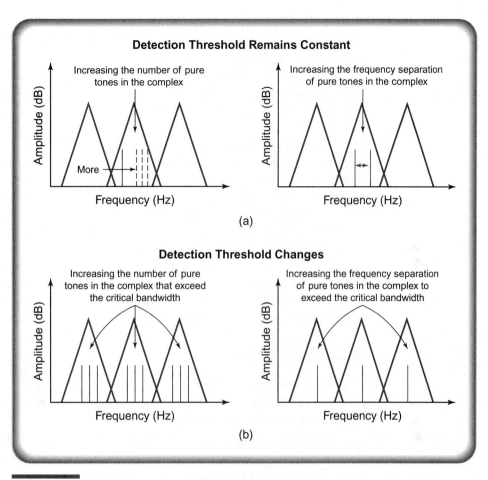

FIGURE 8-11 Thresholds of Complex Tones—A Comparison of Listening Conditions Regarding the Threshold of Multitone Complexes: (a) If, in the presence of three adjacent critical bands, an experimenter either increases the number of pure tone components in the multitone complex or increases the frequency spacing among the components, threshold of the complex does not change as long as all the components in the complex remain within one critical band. (b) The threshold of the multitone complex changes when the number of components in the complex expands, such that they exceed the bandwidth of a single critical band, or when the frequency spacing among the components increases beyond the critical bandwidth. The overall power of the complexes remains constant in both (a) and (b).

regarding the nature, or direction, of the change in detection. Gassler's and a more recent study by Higgens and Turner (1990) suggest that detection thresholds of the periodic complexes increase as the frequency spacing of the individual pure tone components exceed the critical bandwidth. Other experimenters suggest that the threshold of the periodic complex decreases once the frequency components or spacing exceeds the critical bandwidth (Buus, Musch, and Florentine, 1998; Green, 1958). This would suggest that the energy in adjacent critical bands summate to aid in detection. For our purposes, however, it doesn't matter whether audibility improves or worsens as the stimulus's spectral range widens. What is important is that there appears to be a *change* in detection threshold once the individual pure tones within the complex exceed the bandwidth of the critical band.

Figure 8-11 attempts to summarize these findings. In the top panel, either adding more pure tone components to the signal *or* increasing the frequency separation between two components results in fixed detection ability, as long as the pure tone components lie within a single critical band. In the bottom panel, either adding more pure tone components to the signal *or* increasing the frequency separation between a multi-component pure tone complex changes detection ability once the spectral energy exceeds the bandwidth of a single critical band. Whether audibility improves or worsens, at this point, doesn't really matter. The important conclusion is that it changes, suggesting that spectral processing is altered once the complex signal spills into adjacent critical bands. This provides further support for the existence of the critical bands.

■ CHAPTER SUMMARY

We have covered many important concepts related to the frequency selectivity of the inner ear and the critical band. After reading and studying this chapter, you should be able to do the following:

- Explain how the concept of critical bands helps us to understand the empirical evidence regarding the masking behaviors of pure tones, wideband noise, and narrow-band noise on pure tone signals.

- Relate the concept of critical bands to electronic filters.

- Discuss the function and purpose of high-pass, low-pass, and band-pass filters.

- Identify the important spectral characteristics of high-pass, low-pass, and band-pass filters.

- Outline the basic principles and assumptions of the critical band theory as presented by Fletcher.

- Describe Fletcher's masking study and explain how it supports the existence of the critical bands and illustrates the important filtering characteristics of the cochlea.

- Summarize the relationship between the frequency selectivity of the critical bands and signal frequency, as reported by Fletcher and later investigations.

- Define loudness summation and how this phenomenon supports the existence of the critical bands.

- Describe our perceptions of complex periodic sounds as a function of tonal separation and explain how the critical band theory supports the experimental evidence regarding the audibility of these sounds.

■ REFERENCES

Buus, S., and H. Musch. "On Loudness at Threshold." *Journal of the Acoustical Society of America* 104 (1998): 399–409.

Feldtkeller, R., and E. Zwicker. *Das Ohr als Nachrichtenempfanger.* Stuttgart, Germany: S. Hirzel, 1956.

Fletcher, H. "Auditory Patterns." *Review Modern Physics* 12 (1940): 47–65.

Gassler, G. "Über die Horschwelle für Schallereignisse mit verschieden breitem Frequenzspektrum." *Acustica* 4 (1954): 408–414.

Green, D. M. "Detection of Multiple Component Signals in Noise." *Journal of the Acoustical Society of America* 30, 10 (1958): 904–911.

Greenwood, D. D. "Critical Bandwidth and the Frequency Coordinates of the Basilar Membrane." *Journal of the Acoustical Society of America* 33 (1961): 1344–1356.

Hawkins, J. E., and S. S. Stevens. "The Masking of Pure Tones and of Speech by White Noise." *Journal of the Acoustical Society of America* 22 (1950): 6–13.

Higgens, M. B., and C. W. Turner. "Summation Bandwidths at Threshold in Normal and Hearing-Impaired Listeners." *Journal of the Acoustical Society of America* 88 (1990): 2625–2630.

Kiang, N.Y.-S., T. Watanabe, E. C. Thomas, and L. F. Clark. *Discharge Patterns of Single Fibers in the Cat's Auditory Nerve.* Cambridge, MA: MIT Press, 1965.

Scharf, B. "Complex Sounds and Critical Bands." *Psychology Bulletin* 58 (1961): 205–217.

Scharf, B. "Critical Bands." In *Foundations of Modern Auditory Theory,* vol. I, edited by J. V. Tobias, 157–202. New York: Academic Press, 1970.

von Bekesy, G. *Experiments in Hearing.* New York: McGraw-Hill, 1960.

Wegel, R. L., and C. E. Lane, C. E. "The Auditory Masking of One Pure Tone by Another and Its Probable Relation to the Dynamics of the Inner Ear." *Physics Review* 23 (1924): 266–285.

Zwicker, E., G. Flottorp, and S. S. Stevens, S. S. "Critical Bandwidth in Loudness Summation." *Journal of the Acoustical Society of America* 29 (1957): 548–557.

9

FREQUENCY DISCRIMINATION

◼ OVERVIEW

In this chapter, we explore the empirical evidence regarding our discrimination ability for frequency. In other words, if we are presented with a pure tone at 1,000 Hz, how different does a second pure tone have to be, in frequency, for us to judge the tones as being different? What is our discrimination threshold for frequency? Does our ability change with the frequency of the first pure tone? The question is whether the differential thresholds for frequency are constant for frequencies throughout the audible spectrum or increase or decrease as frequency changes. Do the intensities of the tones matter? Is our frequency discrimination ability better or poorer for high-intensity versus low-intensity sounds? These are some of the questions we answer in this chapter.

The approach in this chapter very much parallels that in Chapter 6. You may want to look back at Chapter 6 and refamiliarize yourself with the general concepts of discrimination thresholds and the experimental paradigm used to measure them. In this chapter, as was the case for intensity discrimination thresholds, we review experimental evidence concerning our discrimination ability for frequency as a function of frequency and as a function of intensity. We relate these findings to the critical band. Finally, we see how well Weber's law predicts our frequency discrimination ability.

◼ MEASURING FREQUENCY DISCRIMINATION

The **method of constant stimuli**, as applied to the measurement of **frequency discrimination thresholds**, is illustrated in Figure 9-1. Recall that this psychophysical method is sometimes used to measure thresholds of discrimination; the listener is presented with a standard stimulus, followed by a variable stimulus. The experimenter fixes the standard stimulus's intensity and frequency, which never change throughout the listening trials. The experimenter also sets the intensity of the variable stimulus, and, because we are interested in frequency discrimination ability, the variable intensity is always the same as the standard intensity. The experimenter chooses the frequency of the variable stimulus, and it usually represents five to seven different pure tone frequencies. Typically, one of the five to seven pure tones equals the frequency of the standard stimulus.

During each listening trial, the subject is presented the standard stimulus, followed by the variable stimulus, with a silent interval between them. One of the variable pure tones is chosen randomly to pair with the standard. The listener is required to judge the second stimulus as being higher in pitch than the standard. This is a two-alternative forced-choice procedure; the listener needs to determine whether the second sound is higher in pitch than the first—yes or no. Likewise, the experimenter may choose to have the listener make judgments as to whether the variable stimulus is lower in pitch than the standard. Again, the listener must make a yes-or-no decision for each trial.

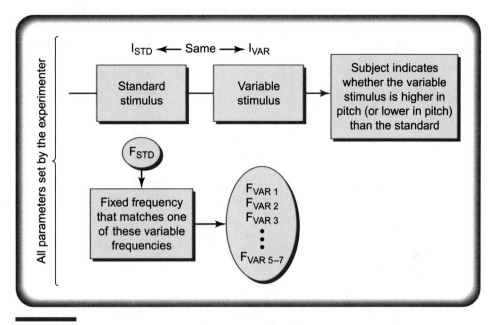

FIGURE 9-1 Experimental Paradigm for the Measurement of Frequency Discrimination Thresholds Using the Method of Constant Stimuli—The Typical Parameters Involved in Measuring Differential Thresholds for Frequency Using the Method of Constant Stimuli: A standard stimulus, whose frequency (F_{STD}) and intensity (I_{STD}) are set by the experimenter, is followed by a variable stimulus, which shares the same intensity (I_{VAR}) as the standard stimulus. The frequency of the variable stimulus (F_{VAR}) is randomly selected from five to seven values predetermined by the experimenter. Usually, one of the variable frequencies matches the standard frequency. The listener must judge whether the variable stimulus is higher (or lower) in pitch, compared to the standard.

The listening trials continue in this manner until each of the variable frequencies has been paired many times with the fixed standard, with the experimenter keeping track of the listener's judgments. Once each variable frequency has been paired with the standard many times, the experimenter represents the results in terms of a **psychometric function**.

The psychometric function illustrated in Figure 9-2 plots the percentage of times the listener judged the variable stimulus higher in pitch than the standard over all the listening trials, as a function of the different frequency values of the variable stimulus. In this hypothetical example, as the frequency of the variable increases, the percentage of times it is judged higher in pitch than the standard increases as well.

To estimate the **frequency difference limen**:

- The 75 percent performance point is found along the ordinate and carried over until it intersects with the psychometric function.

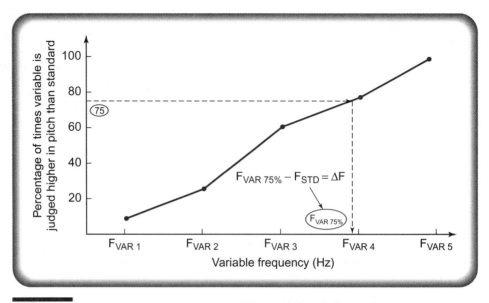

FIGURE 9-2 Determining Frequency Discrimination Threshold from the Psychometric Function—Results of a Hypothetical Frequency Discrimination Study Employing the Method of Constant Stimuli: The percentage of times the listener judged the variable stimulus to be higher in pitch than the standard is plotted as a function of the variable frequency. The variable frequency corresponding to 75% performance is interpolated and subtracted from the frequency of the standard. This difference is the discrimination threshold for frequency at the frequency and presentation level of the standard stimulus.

- The frequency of the variable corresponding to this performance level is interpolated from the abscissa.
- Finally, the difference between the frequency of the variable stimulus corresponding to 75 percent performance and the frequency of the standard is calculated and taken as the **discrimination threshold** (ΔF, expressed in hertz) for sounds at the frequency and intensity of the standard stimulus. See Figure 9-2 for a summary of this process.

The magnitude of ΔF is interpreted much the same way as values of ΔI.

- A relatively large magnitude of ΔF suggests *poor* discrimination performance. Poor frequency discrimination suggests that the listener needs a larger frequency separation between two tones to judge them as different.
- A relatively small magnitude of ΔF suggests *better* discrimination performance. Better discrimination means that the listener needs a smaller acoustic difference between two sounds, in this case in terms of frequency, to reliably judge the sounds as being different.

Lastly, because we are dealing with frequency discrimination ability, hearing scientists tend to view the magnitude of ΔF values as indicative of the relative degree of **tuning** or **frequency selectivity** of the ear.

- Listening conditions that bring about relatively large values of ΔF suggest relatively poor tuning or frequency selectivity of the ear.

- Conditions that result in relatively small values of ΔF suggest sharper tuning and more frequency selectivity.

FREQUENCY DISCRIMINATION AS A FUNCTION OF SIGNAL FREQUENCY

Figure 9-3 illustrates typical results from a frequency discrimination study using a method of constant stimuli paradigm. Reported by Small and Brandt (1963), discrimination thresholds from normal-hearing listeners are plotted as a function

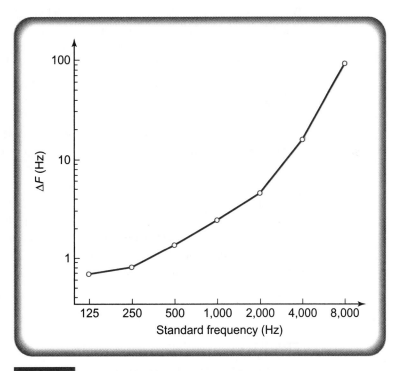

FIGURE 9-3 Frequency Discrimination Thresholds as a Function of Frequency: Average frequency discrimination threshold (ΔF) values are plotted as a function of frequency. The presentation level of the pure tone signals was 40 dB SL. The method of constant stimuli was used to determine the discrimination thresholds. (After Small and Brandt, 1963, from Small, 1973.)

of (standard) pure tone frequency. The intensity of the standard and the variable stimulus was 40 dB SL. Figure 9-3 indicates that, as the frequency of the standard signal increases from 125 Hz through 8,000 Hz, discrimination thresholds for frequency increase. This finding suggests that, for lower-frequency sounds, listeners can judge pitch or frequency differences more reliably at smaller frequency separations, compared to higher-frequency tones, where a greater difference in frequency is needed. In other words, the frequency selectivity, or tuning, of the ear becomes progressively *poorer* as the overall frequency of the sounds get higher.

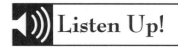

AN EARLY STUDY OF FREQUENCY DISCRIMINATION

Over the years, the experimental paradigm used for measuring normal human discrimination thresholds for frequency has varied to include psychophysical methods other than the method of constant stimuli. An early report by Shower and Biddulph (1931) is considered the classic study in the area of frequency discrimination ability. These researchers at Bell Laboratories presented their listeners with a complex signal that modulated, or changed, its frequency about three times each second. The frequency separation between the higher and lower frequencies was gradually increased, and listeners were required to indicate when they were just able to perceive the frequency change. While this study is widely cited as the gold standard for our empirical evidence regarding frequency discrimination ability, the stimuli ultimately presented to their subjects consisted of a very complex spectrum due to the changes in frequency over time. This aspect compromised the validity of their study, in that auditory perceptions other than frequency discrimination may have occurred, adding additional error to their observations. While the overall trend of the effect of frequency on frequency discrimination reported by Shower and Biddulph is upheld today, their results contain a significant amount of inaccuracy compared to more recent investigations, especially for low-frequency signals (Harris, 1952).

FREQUENCY DISCRIMINATION AND THE CRITICAL BAND

Given that frequency discrimination thresholds increase in magnitude as the frequency of the standard stimulus increases, at least for pure tones of moderate intensity, how does this finding compare to what we have learned about the frequency selectivity characteristics of the critical band hypothesis? Actually, the question is not quite right, in an historical sense because Fletcher's model of the critical bands was developed to help explain the empirical masking evidence of the day, as well as frequency discrimination ability and its relationship to stimulus frequency. Shower and Biddulph's data, although later shown to be somewhat inaccurate, was known to Fletcher at the time he published his renowned paper on auditory patterns. So the question really should be how does the critical band concept take into account and explain the empirical evidence of frequency discrimination like those shown in Figure 9-3?

Remember that Fletcher (1940) hypothesized and provided evidence that the bandwidth of the critical bands widen as the center frequency of the band increases. Along the length of the basilar membrane from base to apex, the center frequency of the critical bands decreases, going from high to low frequency, and the bandwidth of the critical bands narrows. The critical band concept assumes that, for a listener to judge two pure tones as being different in terms of frequency, the tones must be processed in separate critical bands; that is, their frequency separation must be enough that they fall, at a minimum, into adjacent critical bands, not within the same critical band. Empirical evidence supports the notion that the bandwidth of the critical bands is wider at the base of the cochlea, where high-frequency sounds are represented. Therefore, a greater degree of frequency separation must exist between two pure tones at the basal end of the cochlea to get them into separate critical bands, a conclusion that accounts for the larger ΔF values for higher-frequency tones. Likewise, because the bandwidth of the critical bands decreases toward the apex of the cochlea, the frequency separation between two pure tones can become less and still get the signals into separate critical bands. We see empirical evidence that the magnitude of ΔF becomes progressively smaller as the frequency of the tones is reduced.

Figure 9-4 illustrates this reasoning. The figure shows a pair of adjacent critical bands at each end of the cochlea. The first pair (two low-frequency pure tones) represent the apical end of the cochlea where the bandwidths of the critical bands are relatively narrow. The second pair (two high-frequency pure tones) represent the basal end of the cochlea where the critical bands have wider bandwidths. Four separate pure tones fall within the centers of the four critical bands. The frequency separation (ΔF) of the tones at the apical end (low frequencies) is different from the frequency separation (ΔF) of the tone pair at the basal end (high frequencies) of the cochlea. Smaller physical separation between the tones is required for the apical end than for the basal end in order to get the tones into adjacent critical bands. Therefore, we would correctly predict that ΔF *increases* as overall frequency increases.

FREQUENCY DISCRIMINATION AND WEBER'S LAW

Weber's law states the relationship of stimulus discrimination and stimulus magnitude:

$$\frac{\Delta S}{S} = \textbf{constant}$$

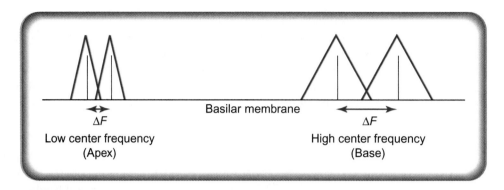

FIGURE 9-4 Explanation of Increasing Frequency Discrimination Thresholds with Frequency Using the Critical Band Model: Schematic of the basilar membrane, unrolled, illustrating two pairs of adjacent critical bands at either end of the cochlea. Vertical lines within the center of each of the four critical bands represent pure tones at the limits of frequency discrimination (ΔF) in the adjacent critical band pair. Because the bandwidth of the critical bands at the basal end of the basilar membrane is wider, a greater frequency separation between the two pure tones (ΔF) is necessary for the listener to judge them as being different. Likewise, because the bandwidth of the critical bands at the apical end of the cochlea is narrower, the frequency spacing between two pure tones in adjacent critical bands can be reduced for the listener to judge them as different.

In Chapter 6, we saw that this hypothesis seriously underestimates the empirical evidence on intensity discrimination ability, which in fact suggests the opposite relationship between intensity discrimination thresholds and stimulus intensity. Discrimination thresholds for intensity are shown to decrease as stimulus intensity increases for sounds close to threshold. For sounds moderately and significantly above threshold, discrimination thresholds for intensity remain relatively constant.

In the case of frequency discrimination, the question is whether Weber's law is a reasonable predictor of the empirical evidence on our discrimination ability for frequency. In a word, yes, it is, inasmuch as ΔF is changing in the right direction as frequency increases. Weber's law predicts that ΔF increases with increasing frequency (F) for the fraction to remain constant, which it does based on the empirical evidence. So it would appear that, although Weber's law seriously underestimates our discrimination ability for intensity, it does a better job of predicting our frequency discrimination ability.

In summary, empirical evidence suggests that differential thresholds of frequency sensitivity increase as frequency increases. The frequency separation required between two pure tones to be judged as different increases as we travel from the apex to the base of the basilar membrane. The frequency selectivity of the ear becomes better as we move from the base to the apex of the cochlea. This observation corresponds favorably with the hypothesis that the bandwidths of the critical bands increase as we move from those characterized by low center frequency (at the apical end of the cochlea) to those characterized by high center frequency (at the basal end of the cochlea). This observation also suggests that Weber's law does a better job of predicting frequency discrimination ability than it does predicting intensity discrimination ability.

■ FREQUENCY DISCRIMINATION AS A FUNCTION OF INTENSITY

So far we have seen evidence of our frequency discrimination ability only for sounds moderately above threshold, not for pure tones that are either very close to threshold or very much above it. The question is whether our ability to judge frequency differences between two sounds depend on their overall intensity. In other words, does ΔF increase, decrease, or remain constant for soft sounds, moderate sounds, and loud sounds?

Figure 9-5 helps us answer this question. This figure presents data from Shower and Biddulph. Plotted are Weber's fractions ($\Delta F/F$) as a function of stimulus intensity, in decibels sensation level. The Weber fraction, rather than the raw ΔF values, is represented on the ordinate to take into account the fact that frequency discrimination thresholds are different for different frequencies. Plotting the Weber fraction rather than the absolute discrimination threshold allows us to directly compare the effect of intensity on frequency discrimination ability across a wide range of frequencies. Even though Shower and Biddulph didn't employ the psychophysical method of constant stimuli in their experimental paradigm, you can think of the intensity plotted on the abscissa as the standard's stimulus intensity. Remember also that the intensity of the standard and variable stimulus in the method of constant stimuli for frequency discrimination estimation is the same. The parameter of the graph is the frequency of the pure tones. Again, relating this to the method of constant stimuli, you can think of this as the frequency of the standard stimulus.

Figure 9-5 clearly shows that, regardless of the frequency of the standard, the Weber fraction remains constant throughout a broad range of presentation levels. Once the standard and variable tones are presented 15–20 dB above threshold, further increases in stimulus intensity results in no change in frequency discrimination ability. So stimulus intensity does not seem to be an important stimulus variable in our overall frequency discrimination ability, at least for somewhat soft sound through very loud sounds.

This is not to say, however, that intensity plays no role in our frequency discrimination ability. Some functions in Figure 9-5 suggest that, when sounds are very close to threshold (0–10 dB SL), frequency discrimination thresholds are relatively large, particularly for very low-frequency tones (125 Hz and 250 Hz).

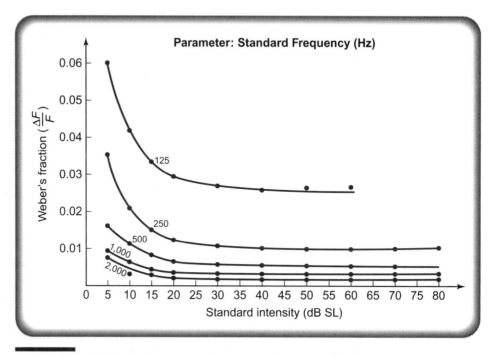

FIGURE 9-5 Weber's Fraction for Frequency as a Function of Signal Presentation Level and Signal Frequency: Frequency discrimination data from Shower and Biddulph (1931) are represented to show the effect of stimulus presentation level and stimulus frequency on differential thresholds for frequency. The Weber fraction is plotted, rather than ΔF, to allow comparison of the effect of intensity at different pure tone frequencies. (After Shower and Biddulph, 1931, from Small, 1973.)

This finding suggests that, when the audibility of the two tones presented to listeners is very poor, the listeners require more frequency separation between them to reliably judge them as being different. Once the audibility of the tones improves, the frequency separation required for discrimination threshold decreases. Recall from Chapter 6 the similar trend regarding intensity discrimination thresholds as a function of overall stimulus intensity. When two tones are presented at intensities very close to threshold, the intensity difference needed for the listeners to reliably judge them as being different is relatively large. Once the audibility of the tones improves, the discrimination thresholds for intensity decrease. Therefore, presentation level appears to show the same effect for both frequency and intensity discrimination. For sounds that are clearly audible, a further increase in stimulus intensity does not significantly alter discrimination ability, for better or worse. On the other hand, when sounds are very close to detection threshold, discrimination ability suffers to some extent.

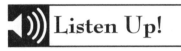 **Listen Up!**

BE CAREFUL WITH FIGURE 9-5

Although the discussion of the effect of stimulus intensity on frequency discrimination is generally accurate, we need to be cautious with our interpretations of Figure 9-5. The effect of presentation level on frequency discrimination that we see from Shower and Biddulph seems especially significant for the low-frequency sounds. However, because of the temporal characteristics of the stimuli used in their study to estimate frequency discrimination thresholds, data regarding these low-frequency sounds are especially suspect (Harris, 1952). Therefore, the effect of presentation level on frequency discrimination, especially for 125 Hz and 250 Hz, may be overestimated in Figure 9-5.

In summary, our ability to discriminate frequency differences between pure tones agrees well with the empirical evidence of the masking effects of pure tones and on the general assumptions made by the critical band theory. Namely, our discrimination ability for frequency is not the same at the two ends of the cochlea. At the base of the cochlea, where high-frequency sounds are represented, the magnitude of frequency discrimination thresholds is relatively large. At the apex of the cochlea, where low-frequency sounds are represented, ΔF values are much smaller. Indeed, empirical evidence suggests that the bandwidths of the critical bands become narrower as we move from the base to the apex of the basilar membrane.

The effect of presentation level on frequency discrimination appears similar to its effect on intensity discrimination. Specifically, for sounds that are audible, as presentation level is increased, frequency discrimination ability remains constant. Only when sounds approach absolute threshold values do we see presentation level influencing our discrimination ability. As sounds become increasingly less audible—close to absolute thresholds for detection—frequency discrimination ability becomes poorer. We saw evidence of this same effect of presentation level on intensity discrimination ability.

Finally, the ability of Weber's law to adequately match empirical evidence regarding our frequency discrimination threshold as a function of frequency allows us to compare our discrimination ability for frequency with our discrimination ability for intensity. Weber's law reasonably predicts the change in discrimination thresholds for frequency with increasing frequency. For the Weber fraction to remain constant, ΔF must increase with increasing frequency. Empirical evidence indicates that this is the case. Although Weber's law is not a perfect predictor of human frequency discrimination ability, it is in the right direction. So we can conclude that, although our ability to discriminate differences in the frequency between two sounds is good, it's not nearly as keen as our ability to discriminate differences in intensity between two sounds. This assumption is based on the fact that Weber's law somewhat predicts the change in frequency discrimination ability with frequency but seriously underestimates the change in intensity discrimination with intensity, especially at high levels. As stated in Chapter 6, our auditory system is exquisitely designed to detect very small intensity changes to a sound. This is not to say that our frequency discrimination ability is poor. On the contrary, our frequency discrimination ability is very good; it's just that our intensity discrimination ability is much better over a wider range of stimulus intensities.

■ CHAPTER SUMMARY

We have covered several important concepts related to normal human discrimination ability for frequency. After reading and studying this chapter, you should be able to do the following:

- Relate the concept of discrimination thresholds for frequency to discrimination thresholds for intensity, explain the auditory skill involved with these thresholds, and describe how the skill for discrimination threshold for frequency is similar to that for discrimination threshold for intensity.

- Outline the psychophysical method of constant stimuli procedure as it is used to measure the auditory discrimination threshold for frequency.

- Calculate the frequency discrimination threshold from a psychometric function generated from a listener.

- Describe the role of stimulus frequency on our ability to discriminate frequency differences between pure tones.

- Explain how the experimental evidence on our ability to discriminate frequency differences between pure tones provides support for the critical band theory in general and corroborates empirical evidence regarding the bandwidth of the critical bands at different ends of the cochlea in particular.

- Describe the role of stimulus intensity on our ability to discriminate frequency differences between pure tones.

- Describe the ability of Weber's law to predict auditory frequency discrimination ability and explain how the empirical evidence from Small and Brandt, for instance, provides support for your statements regarding the accuracy of Weber's law in predicting differential sensitivity for frequency.

- Compare our overall ability to discriminate frequency with our overall ability to discriminate intensity and explain the evidence you use to support your comparison.

■ REFERENCES

Fletcher, H. "Auditory Patterns." *Review Modern Physics* 12 (1940): 47–65.

Harris, J. D. "Pitch Discrimination." *Journal of the Acoustical Society of America* 24 (1952): 750–755.

Shower, E. G., and R. Biddulph. "Differential Pitch Sensitivity of the Ear." *Journal of the Acoustical Society of America* 3 (1931): 275–287.

Small, A. M. "Psychoacoustics." In *Normal Aspects of Speech Hearing and Language*, 1st ed., edited by F. D. Minifie, T. J. Hixon, and F. Williams, 343–420. Upper Saddle River, NJ: Prentice Hall, 1973.

Small, A. M., and J. F. Brandt. "Differential Thresholds for Frequency." *Journal of the Acoustical Society of America* 35 (1963): 787.

10

PITCH PERCEPTION

The important concepts you will learn in this chapter are:

- The definition of pitch.
- The effect of stimulus frequency on pitch perception.
- Direct and indirect procedures used by hearing scientists to obtain estimates of pitch from human listeners.
- The effect of stimulus intensity on pitch perception.
- The unit of pitch estimation.
- Equal pitch contours.
- Historical context and the basic premise of the place theory of pitch perception and of the volley theory of pitch perception.
- Models used to explain our perception of pitch for simple and complex sounds.
- The case of the missing fundamental.
- Periodicity pitch.
- A modern-day theory of pitch perception.

Case of the Missing Fundamental

Classical Theory/ Place Theory of Pitch Perception

Direct Magnitude Estimation

Direct Procedures of Pitch Estimation

Equal Pitch Contours

Harmonic

Indirect Procedure of Pitch Estimation

Indirect Procedures of Pitch Perception

Mel

Periodicity Pitch

Phase Locking

Pitch

Pitch Matching

Tonotopic Organization

Volley Theory/Rate Theory of Pitch Perception

■ OVERVIEW

Not long ago, auditory theory was primarily related to theories of pitch perception (Tobias, 1970). Investigations into which acoustic parameters determine our sense of pitch, along with theories to explain our perceptions, have dominated the interest of hearing scientists for many years. **Pitch** is the part of our auditory perception primarily related to the frequency of a pure tone. It is a psychological perception, like loudness, that can't be measured directly. In addition, the acoustic parameters of a stimulus other than frequency can influence our perception of pitch. Previous studies regarding our pitch perception have led to the development of several theories about how we determine the pitch of a certain sound. In this chapter, we examine

- Important acoustic parameters that influence our pitch perception.
- The experimental methods hearing scientists use to estimate pitch.
- A historical approach regarding theories of pitch perception.

■ STIMULUS FREQUENCY AND ITS EFFECT ON PITCH

The frequency of a sound is directly related to its pitch. For example, on a piano, as you play the keys from left to right, the pitch of the notes increases, as well as the primary frequency of the piano string vibrations. Tuning forks, as they change in size from large to small, increase their rate of vibration and bring about an increase in the pitch that we perceive. Although frequency and pitch appear to be directly related, in that an increase in one brings about an increase in the other, the question is whether the relationship is linear. In Chapter 5, we learned that intensity and loudness are linearly related, at least for narrow bands of noise and some pure tones. An increase in the intensity of a sound results in a proportional increase in its perceived loudness. Does the same hold true for frequency and pitch? The results of a 1963 study provide an answer to this question.

In that year, Beck and Shaw reported results of a pitch estimation study using over 600 young adult listeners. The subjects were presented with the experimental listening paradigm illustrated in Figure 10-1. A standard stimulus, a 523-Hz pure tone delivered at a sound pressure level equivalent to a loudness of 20 sones, was followed by a variable pure tone. The variable tone was also adjusted to an intensity equivalent to a loudness of 20 sones and to one of six pure tone frequencies ranging from 131 Hz to 4,186 Hz. The experimenters preselected the six variable pure tone frequencies. The subjects were told to assign the pitch of the standard tone a value of 100 and then to provide a numerical value of the pitch of the variable tone, based on the 100-unit standard pitch. For example, if the listener thought the pitch of the variable was twice as high as the standard,

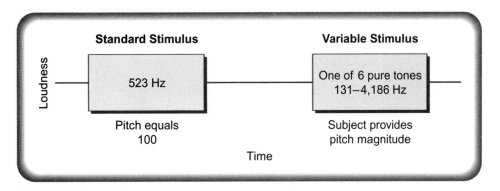

FIGURE 10-1 Stimulus Paradigm for the Estimation of Pitch Using a Direct Magnitude Estimation Procedure: This is the experimental paradigm employed by Beck and Shaw (1963) to measure the effect of stimulus frequency on pitch.

the assigned value would be 200. If the listener thought the pitch of the variable was lower than the standard, the value would be less than 100. This experimental paradigm is an example of a **direct procedure of pitch estimation**. Specifically, it is a **direct magnitude estimation** procedure for pitch, very similar to the experimental paradigm described in Figure 5-1, which was the direct magnitude estimation for loudness procedure employed by Stevens and Tulving (1957). Estimating perceptions of pitch and loudness, as we will soon see, have very similar approaches.

Beck and Shaw's results are shown in Figure 10-2. The average magnitude estimation of pitch, based on 100, is plotted as a function of the six different frequencies of the variable pure tone. The frequency of the standard pure tone (523 Hz) is also indicated in the figure. We can see from the figure that, as the frequency of the variable pure tones increased from 131 Hz to 4,186 Hz, the average pitch estimates increase from about 30 to almost 400. This function clearly indicates a *direct relationship* between stimulus frequency and pitch. As the frequency of the variable tone increases, the magnitude of pitch estimation increases as well. The relationship, however, is *not linear*. The function shown in Figure 10-2 cannot be described as a straight line. An increase in the frequency of a pure tone does not result in a proportional increase in the magnitude of its pitch estimation. This is one important difference between the relationship of stimulus intensity and loudness versus stimulus frequency and pitch. Intensity and loudness are linearly related; frequency and pitch are not.

Studies prior to Beck and Shaw's also reported a direct, nonlinear relationship between stimulus frequency and pitch estimation (Stevens and Volkmann, 1940; Stevens, Volkmann, and Newman, 1937). While the slope of the functions relating stimulus frequency and the magnitude of pitch estimation varies among these

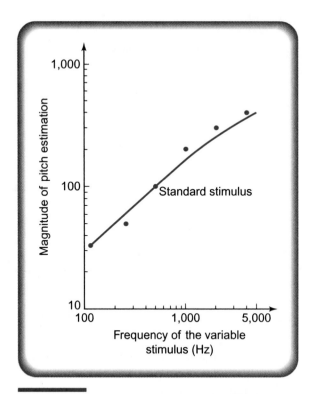

FIGURE 10-2 The Relationship Between Stimulus
Frequency and Pitch: Direct estimates
of pitch magnitude are plotted as a
function of stimulus frequency. (After
Beck and Shaw, 1963, from Small, 1973.)

studies, the relationship between frequency and pitch has always been shown to be
direct and nonlinear. To paraphrase Stevens and Volkmann, pitch is not the same
as frequency, but pitch is a function of frequency.

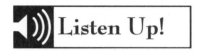 Listen Up!

VARIABILITY OF PITCH ESTIMATES

The relationship between frequency and pitch has long been difficult for hearing scientists
and musicians alike to sort out. Pitch scaling procedures appear to result in more listener
variability than is inherent in loudness estimation. Although the relationship between frequency and pitch has always been shown to be direct, the nature of the function of this
relationship can vary significantly depending on the frequency of the standard tone (Beck
and Shaw, 1963) and on whether a small number of subjects are making numerous estimations of pitch versus a large number of listeners making one or two pitch estimations (Beck

and Shaw, 1963). Although both loudness and pitch are psychological attributes we give to a sound, and although estimates of each are obtained from listeners in similar ways, pitch estimation appears to vary more across listeners and across experimental listening conditions, compared to loudness.

STIMULUS INTENSITY AND ITS EFFECT ON PITCH

It's been emphasized many times throughout this text that the acoustic parameters we use to measure the physical dimensions of a sound (frequency, intensity, duration) should never be confused with or used to define the psychological perceptions we may experience. So, although stimulus intensity is very important in determining our loudness perception and stimulus frequency has a significant effect regarding our pitch perception, they are not the only acoustic variables contributing to our perceptions. In Chapter 5, we discovered that the frequency of a pure tone has some influence on our perception of its loudness. Therefore, we should not be at all surprised to learn that stimulus intensity can alter our perception of pitch.

An early and most often cited study exploring the effect of stimulus intensity on pitch perception comes from Snow (1936), who employed a way of estimating pitch perception from his listeners known as **pitch matching**. This is an example of an **indirect procedure of pitch estimation**, much like loudness balance is an indirect procedure for loudness estimation. His experimental procedure answers the question at hand, namely, how much influence does stimulus intensity have on pitch perception?

Snow's experimental procedure is complex and involves a number of different steps to address the effect of intensity on pitch perception. In the first step of his study, he obtained estimations of pitch from nine listeners for a variety of pure tones 40 phons loud. The experimental paradigm for this first step of his experiment is shown in Figure 10-3.

In a number of trials, the listeners were presented with paired pure tones, a standard and a variable.

- In the *first trial*, the *frequency* of the standard tone was set to 100 Hz and its intensity at a loudness equivalent to 40 phons. The intensity of the variable tone, also set by Snow, was equivalent to a loudness of 40 phons, but the frequency of the variable tone was under the listeners' control. The subjects' task was to listen to the standard tone (100 Hz, 40 phons), followed by the variable tone (40 phons), and adjust the *frequency of the variable tone* so that it had equal pitch to the standard. The frequency (in hertz) of the variable tone was recorded once the subject was done matching the pitch of the two tones.

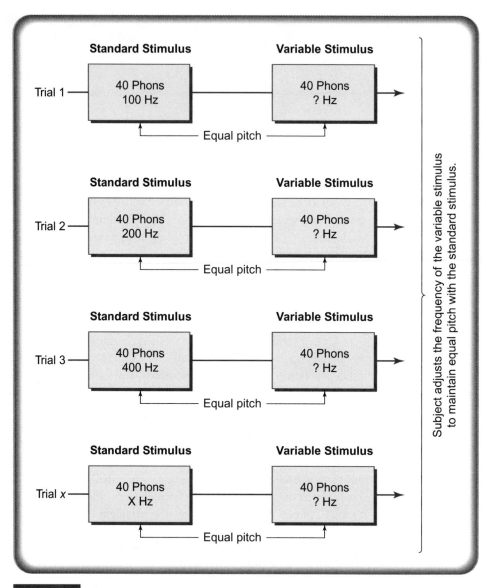

FIGURE 10-3 Step 1 of the Stimulus Paradigm Used in Snow's (1936) Pitch Matching Study: For each listening trial, the subject was required to adjust the frequency of the variable stimulus so that it matched the pitch of the standard tone. All stimuli were presented at a loudness equivalent to 40 phons. The number of listening trials was determined by the number of standard pure tone frequencies investigated by Snow.

- The *second trial* of the first step of Snow's procedure was to change the frequency of the standard tone to 200 Hz, still at 40 phons, and pair it with another variable tone, also at 40 phons. Again, the subjects' task was to adjust the frequency of the variable tone so that it had equal pitch to the standard. Snow recorded the frequency of the variable tone that the listeners ultimately selected.

- In the *third trial*, he presented a standard tone at 400 Hz, 40 phons, and asked the listeners to adjust the frequency of a 40-phon variable tone so that the pitch matched that of the standard. The frequency of the variable tone was recorded, and the listening trials continued to include a wide range of standard pure tone frequencies.

With the paradigm shown in Figure 10-3, the loudness of the standard and variable tones remained the same. Snow chose to equate the loudness of the standard and the variable tones, rather than their physical intensity, because he knew that our sensitivity to pure tones within the frequency range of 100–10,000 Hz varies significantly; so the tones were equated in terms of their relative audibility rather than intensity. Remember that Sivian and White (1933) demonstrated that our sensitivity to very low-frequency pure tones, and to some extent very high-frequency tones, is relatively poor. We are most sensitive to pure tone frequencies between 1,000 Hz and 5,000 Hz.

The second step in Snow's pitch matching paradigm is shown in Figure 10-4. Listeners were again presented with a standard tone followed by a variable tone. As before, Snow preselected the acoustic parameters of the standard tone.

- In the *first trial*, the standard was 100 Hz, 40 phons loud, as in the first trial of the previous step (Figure 10-3). The loudness of the variable tone was also preselected, but this time it had a loudness equivalent to 60 phons. The subjects were instructed to listen to the standard tone, followed by the variable tone, and to adjust the frequency of the variable tone so that its pitch was equal to that of the standard. Keep in mind that the loudness of the standard and variable stimuli is no longer equal. The listeners were instructed to ignore the difference in loudness while matching the pitch of the two tones. Once the subjects had settled on a variable frequency necessary for equal pitch with the standard tone, this frequency was recorded, and Snow moved to the next trial.

- The *second trial* again paired a 40-phon standard tone with a 60-phon variable tone, but the standard tone frequency was increased to 200 Hz. Again instructed to ignore the loudness differences between the two tones, the listeners had to adjust the frequency of the variable tone so that it had equal pitch to the standard. The variable frequency was noted, and the experiment moved to the third listening trial.

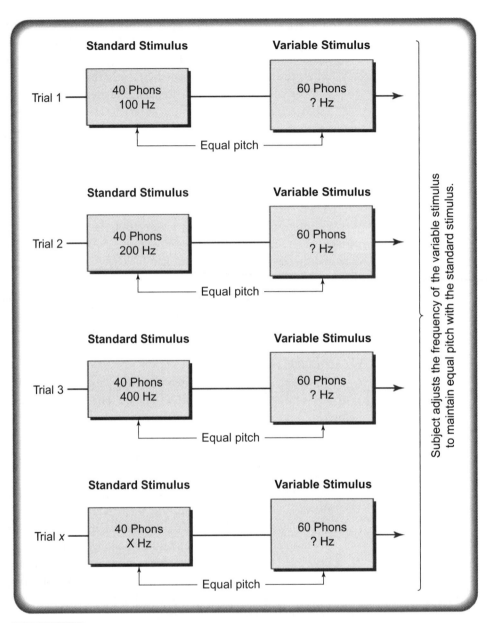

FIGURE 10-4 Step 2 of the Stimulus Paradigm Used in Snow's (1936) Pitch Matching Study: Variable stimuli were presented at an intensity equivalent to a loudness of 60 phons. Standard stimulus remained at 40 phons. For each listening trial, the subject was required to adjust the frequency of the variable stimulus so that it matched the pitch of the standard tone. All stimuli were presented at a loudness equivalent to 40 phons. The number of listening trials was determined by the number of standard pure tone frequencies investigated by Snow.

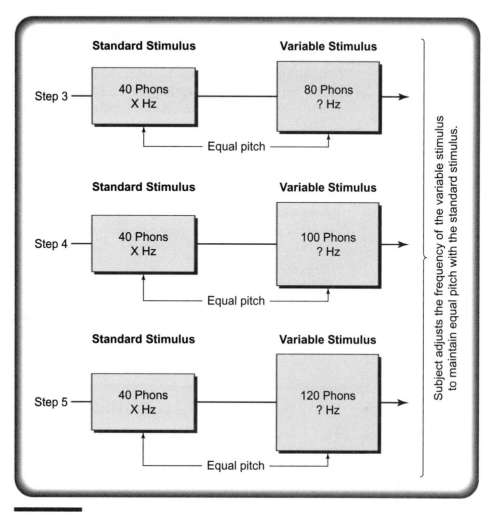

FIGURE 10-5 Steps 3, 4, and 5 of the Stimulus Paradigm Used in Snow's (1936) Pitch Matching Study

- In the *third trial*, the paradigm continued as before, except that the frequency of the standard tone was changed to 400 Hz.

The listening trials continued in this manner, and each time Snow changed the frequency of the standard tone until all the pure tone frequencies of the standard had been investigated.

The remaining steps in Snow's experimental paradigm are illustrated in Figure 10-5. With each step, the loudness of the variable was increased on the order of 20 phons. In each step, the 40-phon standard tone was paired with the louder variable tone. The standard tone took on the frequencies preselected by Snow, each constituting a listening trial and corresponding to the same frequencies as presented in steps 1 and 2. For each listening trial, the subjects were required to adjust the frequency of the louder variable tone to match the pitch of the standard.

Note: As with any field of scientific inquiry, hearing scientists owe a great deal of gratitude to the subjects of their listening experiments, past and present. This experiment had to have been tiresome to sit through! The subjects of any psychoacoustic study, especially older ones, have been extremely important to the contribution of our present-day knowledge regarding auditory perceptions. Long before the days of any sort of review of human subject use, listeners were subjected to, at best, long hours of tedious listening trials and, at worst, exposure to harmful acoustic stimuli.

The results of Snow's study are illustrated in Figure 10-6. Plotted are **equal pitch contours** for the different loudness levels of the variable stimulus as a function of the frequency of the standard stimulus. The frequency values provided by the subjects for the variable stimulus are represented as pitch change (%). In other words, the average variable frequency, as determined by the listeners, to have equal pitch to the standard tone is represented as the *proportion of frequency change*, compared to the frequency of the standard, within the trial. For example, when a 100-Hz, 40-phon standard pure tone is paired with a 100-phon variable tone, the average

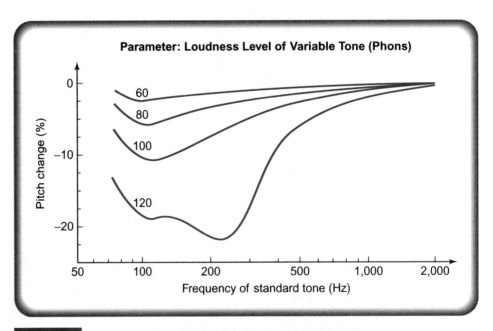

FIGURE 10-6 Equal Pitch Contours: Pitch estimates, represented as pitch change (%) is plotted as a function of standard frequency. The parameter is the loudness of the variable tone. (After Snow, 1936, from Small, 1973.)

frequency of the variable stimulus that the listeners' determined to match the pitch of the standard was 90 Hz. This represents a relative pitch change of -10 percent;

$$\frac{100 \text{ Hz}}{100 \text{ Hz} - 90 \text{ Hz}} \times 100\%$$

In this way, the frequency adjustments provided by the listeners are plotted as a function of the different frequencies of the standard tones explored by Snow. The parameter is the loudness level of the variable stimulus. Remember that the loudness of the *standard stimulus* was always 40 phons.

Each of the four functions represented in Figure 10-6 is an equal pitch contour: All the data points falling along a single function have, by definition, the same pitch, even though the loudness and frequencies of the two tones under comparison (standard and variable) are very different. We interpret these contours much the same way as we interpret the equal loudness contours provided by Fletcher and Munson (1933) in Chapter 5. The psychological perception is held constant while the acoustic parameters of the comparison stimuli change.

With respect to the role that loudness plays regarding changes to our perception of pitch, Snow's results suggest that significant changes in pitch brought about by an increase in loudness is confined to the lower frequencies. For pure tones below about 500 Hz, as the tones get louder, their pitch changes significantly, especially for pure tones between 100 Hz and 300 Hz. For mid-frequency tones (1,000–2,000 Hz), pitch doesn't seem to change significantly as the tones become progressively louder. The pitch change for these mid-frequency tones is close to 0 percent, suggesting that the frequency differences between the standard and variable tones were small, even when the variable stimulus was much louder than the standard. The pitch change for lower-frequency tones, however, is significant as the variable tone increases in loudness. The pitch change grows with increases in loudness of the variable stimulus, such that for a very loud (120-phon), low-frequency tone (250 Hz), the change in pitch due to an increase in intensity is on the order of 22 percent. This means that, compared to a 40-phon, 250-Hz (standard) tone, another (variable) tone at a loudness equivalent to 120 phons must have a frequency of approximately 195 Hz to be judged as equal in pitch.

Another important conclusion from Snow's report is related to the *direction* of the pitch change as loudness increases. In Figure 10-6, where we see a significant pitch change in the standard pure tone frequencies, the direction of the change is negative. The subjects were always adjusting the frequency of the variable tone to a frequency *lower* than the frequency of the standard stimulus to maintain equal pitch. This result suggests that the pitch shift for these loud sounds is lower, rather than higher.

In summary, stimulus intensity plays a limited role regarding our perception of pitch. For soft and moderately loud sounds, as we adjust their loudness within this range, our perception of the pitch of the sound doesn't change very much. For very loud sounds, however, especially for low-frequency pure tones, as loudness grows, pitch appears to shift lower. Loud sounds of frequencies higher than about 500 Hz do not seem to change in pitch as loudness increases further.

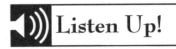

MAGNITUDE OF PITCH SHIFT AND PITCH SHIFT FOR HIGH-FREQUENCY PURE TONES

Further investigation into the pitch change reported by Snow for low-frequency tones has suggested that the magnitude of the pitch change may be overestimated (Cohen, 1961). Hearing scientists agree, however, that the pitch of loud low-frequency tones shifts down; however, the magnitude of the pitch change is disputed. Some evidence suggests that, for pure tones above 2,000 Hz, an increase in loudness brings about an increase in pitch change. In other words, the pitch of higher-frequency pure tones rises as the loudness increases (Small, 1973). This phenomenon is not as well documented as is the pitch shift for loud low-frequency sounds.

COMPARING PITCH ESTIMATION PROCEDURES

When we explained the effect of stimulus frequency and intensity on pitch perception, two different methods for estimating pitch were illustrated:

1. Direct magnitude estimation (DME)

2. Pitch matching

In the case of Beck and Shaw's (1963) study relating the effect of pure tone frequency on pitch perception, a DME procedure was used. Listeners were required to provide a numerical estimation of the pitch of the variable tone, based on the reference (100) defined by the standard tone. As in the case of loudness estimation obtained from DME, the numerical pitch values ultimately provided by the listener reflect a ratio number scale. These values may be added, subtracted, multiplied, and divided with meaning. For example, in the study reported by Beck and Shaw, pure tone frequencies that result in a pitch estimation of 300 by a listener are, by definition, three times higher in pitch than the standard frequency. Likewise, a pitch estimation value of 50 means that the subjects estimated the pitch to be lower than the standard by half. Using a direct pitch estimation procedure, like DME, yields a very powerful pitch measurement scale. If the standard stimulus is a 1,000-Hz pure tone presented with an intensity of 40 dB SL and is assigned a pitch value of 1,000, the unit of the pitch scale is called the **mel**. The pitch of this reference pure tone is equivalent to 1,000 mels. Whenever pitch units are expressed in mels, a direct procedure of pitch estimation, either direct magnitude estimation or direct magnitude production, is implied.

On the other hand, Snow (1936) employed a *pitch matching procedure* as his method of pitch estimation to determine the influence of stimulus intensity on pitch perception. Like loudness balance, pitch matching is an example of an indirect procedure for pitch estimation. Using this procedure, the listener makes decisions only as to whether the two stimuli under comparison are the same, or equal. Therefore, a ratio relationship between the pitch of the stimulus and its frequency is never established. We can compare the frequencies of the standard and the variable only when they have the same pitch, as perceived by the listener. In the case of loudness, you may recall, loudness estimates obtained from loudness balance were expressed in phons. Unfortunately, we have no corollary unit name for pitch values obtained from pitch matching.

Now that we have explored the procedures that hearing scientists use to obtain pitch estimates from listeners and have learned about the role that stimulus frequency and stimulus intensity play in pitch perception, let's turn our attention to how scientists explain our pitch perception. The question is what theory have they developed to explain why and how we assign a certain pitch value to the various sounds we encounter?

■ COMPETING THEORIES OF PITCH PERCEPTION

In the mid-nineteenth century, the beginnings of what would become the basis of two seemingly competing theories of pitch perception emerged.

1. The place theory of pitch perception was formulated by Hermann von Helmholtz in 1863. Certain elements of this theory had been in existence for some time prior to 1863, but Helmholtz is credited for bringing these elements together and presenting them in terms of a scientific theory that could be studied using the scientific method. While some of the specific details of Helmholtz's place theory have turned out to be wrong, its basic premise remains intact today.

2. Volley theory began with a series of acoustic experiments recorded by an obscure scientist named August Seebeck in 1841. Overshadowed by Helmholtz and his place theory for decades, if not for an entire century, elements of a volley theory of pitch perception resurfaced in the twentieth century as neurological investigations of the cochlea proliferated, especially those conducted to obtain neurological responses of the first order auditory neurons of the cochlea.

Our purpose is not to study the history of these theories or their details as they were first developed by Helmholtz and Seebeck. Rather, we concern ourselves with the fundamental premises of the theories as they stand today.

THE PLACE THEORY OF PITCH PERCEPTION

Simply stated, the **place theory of pitch perception**, sometimes referred to as the **classical theory**, maintains that the pitch given to a signal ultimately depends on the *place* along the basilar membrane corresponding to the maximum displacement of the traveling wave response. The tonotopic properties of the traveling wave response is illustrated in Figure 10-7.

- High-frequency sounds entering the cochlea result in a traveling wave response with maximum amplitude occurring near the base of the cochlea.

- Low-frequency sounds result in maximum displacement of the basilar membrane occurring near the apex of the cochlea.

The place theory states that the pitch we ultimately judge for a sound entering the cochlea is determined *only* by the particular place along the length of the basilar membrane that illustrates maximum displacement due to the traveling wave response. Likewise, this theory states that, if the traveling wave response generated from an incoming sound does not result in any significant displacement along some region of the basilar membrane, the pitch of a sound can never match the characteristic frequency of the single auditory neurons innervating that point of the cochlea. The primary basis of the place theory of pitch perception lies with the **tonotopic organization** of the cochlea, both mechanically and neurologically. Place theory is fundamentally a spectral approach to pitch perception.

THE VOLLEY THEORY OF PITCH PERCEPTION

In contrast to the place theory of pitch perception, the **volley theory**, or **rate theory**, maintains that the pitch assigned to a sound relates primarily to the temporal characteristics of the neurological impulses generated by the single-fiber neurons innervating the length of the cochlea. Figure 10-8 provides a very simple schematic of the concept of this theory. At the top of the figure is the waveform of a pure tone, followed by the neurological activity of five hypothetical single auditory fibers responding to the waveform. Each fiber fires at some time during the positive maximum amplitude (condensation) excursion of the waveform. For example, the first fiber responds to the first and eighth waves of condensation of the incoming pure tone. The fifth fiber responds to the fifth and tenth waves. The other fibers respond to other waves of condensation in the ongoing signal. This phenomenon is referred to as the **phase-locking** behavior of single auditory nerve fibers that innervate the length of the cochlea. Its basic premise is that if a single auditory nerve fiber responds to the presence of a pure tone entering the cochlea, it does so only at a time interval corresponding to a point of maximum pressure, or condensation, of the stimulating wave. The nerve fiber matches, or locks, its neurological activity to the phase of the stimulating wave. The basic

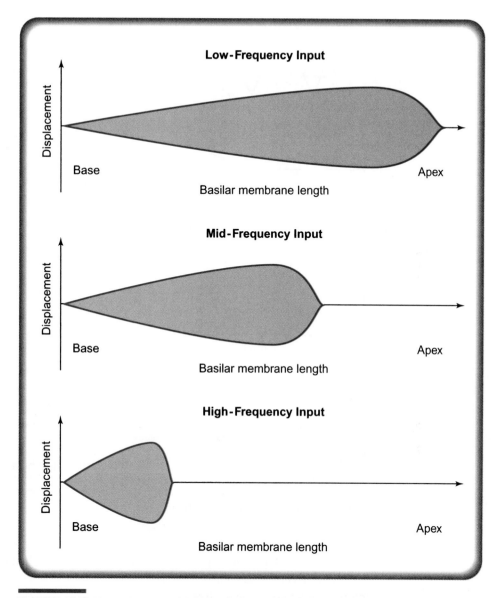

FIGURE 10-7 Place Theory of Pitch Perception: Schematized traveling wave responses to low-, medium-, and high-frequency pure tones. Basilar membrane displacement is represented as a function of distance along the length of the basilar membrane.

premise of the volley theory suggests that when the ear perceives a temporal display of the total amount of neurological activity from all the fibers responding to a pure tone (all five fibers, in Figure 10-8), the pitch assigned equals the rate of combined neurological activity, as represented in the bottom panel of the figure.

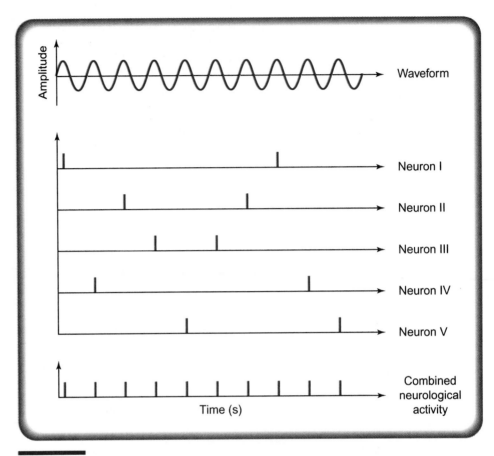

FIGURE 10-8 Volley Theory of Pitch Perception: The waveform of a stimulating pure tone is shown along with the neurological output of five hypothetical single auditory nerve fibers and the combined neurological output of all five fibers as a function of time.

The air pressure change of the pure tone (cycles/s) is coded within the ear in terms of the overall combined neurological activity rate (spikes/s), and the ear uses this information to assign the pitch of the tone.

PLACE THEORY OR VOLLEY THEORY—WHICH IS THE RIGHT ONE?

Although the place and volley theories of pitch perception seem equally logical, they are fundamentally very different.

- Place theory suggests that the most important component to pitch estimation is the exact place along the length of the basilar membrane where maximum physical displacement occurs. It ignores neurological activity from the traveling wave response, beyond the idea that maximum neurological activity is found with the fibers innervating the region of the basilar membrane demonstrating maximum traveling wave displacement. The only important variable is the place of maximum displacement.

- Volley theory essentially ignores the mechanical response of the cochlea in terms of its contribution to pitch estimation. The place where maximum neurological activity occurs is not important. What is important is the time pattern of neurological activity, regardless of where it occurs. Because of the phase-locking behavior of single auditory neurons, the temporal pattern of pressure variation of the input signal is recreated in the temporal pattern of neurological activity, thereby extracting the pitch of the sound.

PITCH PERCEPTION OF SIMPLE SOUNDS

Science can never ultimately prove a theory to be right or wrong, and in this case neither theory is entirely right. What science can do is provide empirical evidence regarding pitch perceptions to various sounds and try to explain these perceptions using one theory or the other. And that is what hearing scientists did, keeping busy with scientific inquiry into pitch perception throughout much of the last century. We now explore some of the empirical evidence reported as a result of their efforts and determine which theory, place or volley, better explains our perceptions.

Perhaps the most fundamental aspect of our auditory behavior related to pitch perception is our ability to discriminate frequency differences between two pure tones. This ability requires us to listen to two pure tones, alike in all respects except their frequency, and judge them as being the same or different. If the frequency difference between the two is such that we hear them as being different, clearly the difference we hear is, in large part, related to the pitch difference.

Hearing scientists typically model our differential thresholds for frequency using excitation patterns. Figure 10-9 illustrates excitation patterns generated from two moderately intense pure tones. The frequency difference between the two pure tones is such that it exceeds our differential threshold for frequency within the frequency region of both tones. This condition suggests that we can consistently hear the pitch difference between these tones.

Based on this display, what landmarks from the excitation patterns might the ear use to distinguish between these tones?

- For one, the ear might look at the frequency separation between the pattern peaks, corresponding to the center frequencies of the critical bands involved in processing the two pure tones. Perhaps, if the frequency separation exceeds a critical amount, this is an indication that the two excitation patterns are different, and we recognize this difference as a pitch difference.

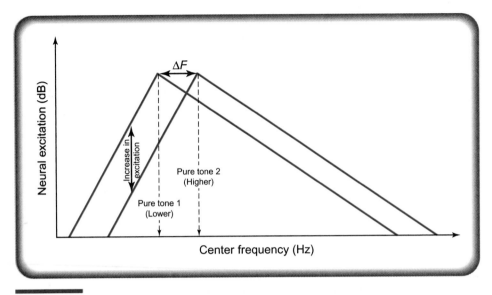

FIGURE 10-9 Excitation Patterns in Response to Two Pure Tones: Excitation patterns of two pure tones are represented as neural excitation as a function of critical band center frequency. The frequency difference between the two tones is such that a pitch difference is noticeable to a listener. Important landmarks that the auditory system might use to recognize the pitch difference are highlighted.

- A second cue might come from the low-frequency sides of both excitation patterns, which are much steeper than the high-frequency sides. If the ear selects a center frequency falling on the low-frequency slope of each excitation pattern, the change in neurological activity at that center frequency, from one pure tone to the next, is significant. Perhaps the ear recognizes the significant change in excitation from one pattern to the other, at this below-peak frequency. This, in turn, is recognized as a pitch difference.

Explaining pitch perception using an excitation pattern model is essentially a place theory of pitch perception. Excitation patterns represent how neurological excitation is distributed along the length of the basilar membrane (a place). The temporal pattern of the neurological activity isn't considered in this model. Given the preceding two important spectral cues concerning significant differences in the excitation patterns of two pure tones with noticeably different pitch, a place theory of pitch perception seems to readily account for our ability to discriminate frequency differences between two pure tones.

There is another auditory phenomenon regarding the pitch shift of a pure tone. See Figure 10-10. Suppose we present a listener with an audible pure tone. The frequency of the tone doesn't matter as long as the tone is audible. A listener

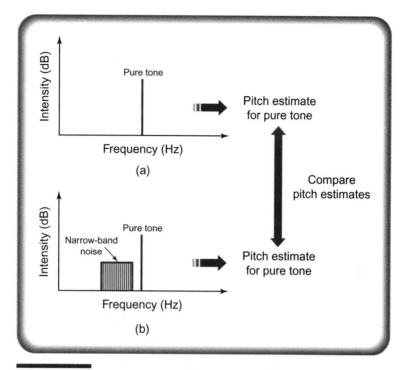

FIGURE 10-10 Pitch Shift of a Pure Tone on the Edge of a Narrow Noise Band: Pitch estimates of a pure tone are obtained in two conditions. (a) The pure tone is presented alone. (b) The pure tone is presented with a narrow band of noise. In comparing the pitch estimates, the pitch of the tone presented simultaneously with the noise is higher.

provides us with an estimation of the pitch of the pure tone, perhaps by employing either a pitch matching procedure or one of the two direct procedures of pitch estimation. Next we deliver this same pure tone to the listener in the presence of a narrow band of noise. The bandwidth of the noise is very narrow, and the intensity of the noise isn't high enough to mask the presence of the noise. In other words, the tone is still audible to the listener even in the presence of the noise. Again, we obtain an estimation of the pitch of the tone.

In Figure 10-10, the frequency of the pure tone is very close to the upper cutoff frequency of the noise. By comparing the pitch estimates of the pure tone in each of the listening conditions, we would discover that they are different. The listener estimates the pitch of the pure tone in the presence of the narrow-band noise *higher* than when the tone is presented in quiet, even though the frequency of the pure tone is the same for the two conditions. Why the pitch of the pure tone changes when presented simultaneously with the narrow-band noise is made clear by comparing the excitation patterns of the pure tone in each condition.

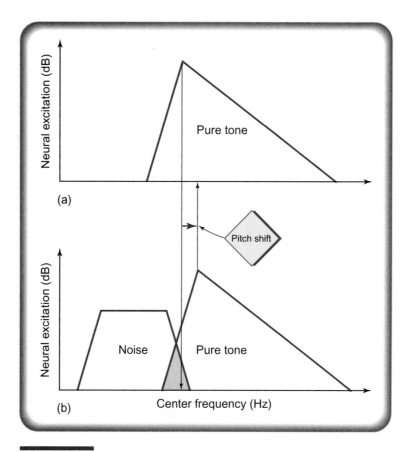

FIGURE 10-11 Using Excitation Patterns to Explain the Pitch Shift of a Pure Tone in the Presence of a Narrow Band of Noise: (a) Excitation patterns for a pure tone alone. (b) Excitation patterns in the presence of a narrow noise band. Because portions of the two excitation patterns overlap, the frequency of the pure tone excitation peak is pushed up. The shift in frequency corresponds to the degree and direction of pitch change.

- In Figure 10-11a, the excitation pattern of the pure tone is presented in quiet. When we obtain a pitch estimation of the single pure tone, the ear is likely determining the center frequency corresponding to the peak amount of excitation from the pattern. Wherever the maximum amount of neurological excitation occurs (the place) is the center frequency corresponding to the pitch.

- Figure 10-11b shows the excitation pattern of the pure tone in the presence of the narrow band of noise. Because the noise is more spectrally complex than the pure tone, it corresponds to a broad area of excitation. Because the tone and the noise are very close to one another, in terms of their place along the length of the basilar membrane where they cause neurological activity, they physically interfere with one another. The upper edge of the noise pattern collides with the lower edge of the tone pattern, as you can see where the two excitation patterns overlap.

As a result of this physical interaction, the peak of the excitation pattern of the pure tone is pushed over a bit to a slightly higher center frequency. As place theory predicts, if we *physically* change the place where maximum excitation occurs, the pitch must change accordingly, and this is precisely what happened to the listener's pitch estimation for the tone. The pitch shifted up to a higher frequency.

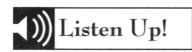 Listen Up!

PITCH SHIFT OF A PURE TONE ON THE LOWER EDGE OF A NARROW-BAND NOISE

If we reverse the spectral relationship between the tone and the noise, the pitch shift occurs in the opposite direction. In other words, if a pure tone frequency is very close to the *lower* cutoff frequency of a narrow-band noise and we compare the pitch estimates for the tone in quiet and in the presence of the noise, the pitch of the tone shifts to a lower frequency. Again, this shift is hypothesized to be due to the physical interaction between the excitation pattern of the noise and the tone, resulting in the peak of the tone excitation pattern moving a little farther down in frequency. This move causes the pitch estimation to move lower, compared to the estimation when the tone is presented alone.

Until now, the place theory of pitch perception seemed to be doing well in providing a reasonable explanation for pitch perception and the changes in pitch we see empirically, using simple sounds like pure tones. A question is whether place theory can account for pitch perception and changes in pitch in more complex auditory stimuli. In the next section, we explore pitch perceptions related to more spectrally and temporally complex stimuli and attempt to determine whether place theory accurately predicts listeners' perceptions.

PITCH PERCEPTION OF COMPLEX SOUNDS

Suppose we were to generate a complex stimulus made up of 11 pure tone frequencies, all 200 Hz apart, with the pure tone amplitudes all equal. The spectrum of such a stimulus is illustrated in Figure 10-12a. The 11 pure tones start at 200 Hz, and each additional pure tone added to the complex increases in frequency by 200 Hz, with the last one 2,200 Hz. We present this complex stimulus to a listener at a comfortable loudness level and ask the subject to provide us with a pitch estimate. The

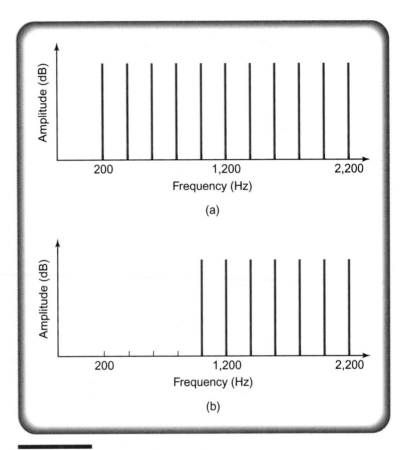

FIGURE 10-12 Multitone Complexes Illustrating the Case of the Missing Fundamental: (a) The stimulus with energy present at the fundamental frequency. (b) The fundamental and the next three pure tone components removed from the stimulus. A listener estimates the pitch of these two stimuli as the same.

listener estimates the pitch of the complex signal to be equal to 200 Hz. According to place theory, the reason has to do with where the maximum amount of spectral energy, or neurological activity, occurs on the basilar membrane. Because the spectrum of this signal contains physical energy at 200 Hz, this explanation appears to be reasonable.

Next, suppose that we filter the complex stimulus, removing the lowest four frequency components. Figure 10-12 illustrates the new, filtered spectrum. The original four pure tone components from 200 Hz through 800 Hz have been removed, leaving a seven-tone complex, the lowest pure tone component at 1,000 Hz and the highest at 2,200 Hz. The frequency separation between the remaining pure tone components is still 200 Hz. The listener again provides an estimate of the pitch of the complex sound. Place theory would predict the pitch to change because, with the new filtered complex, there is no more spectral energy remaining at 200 Hz. In fact, there is no spectral energy below 1,000 Hz. If there is no energy in the spectrum at 200 Hz, the point of maximum displacement of the resulting traveling wave can no longer remain at 200 Hz. The place of maximum excitation must move to a different place on the basilar membrane, and the pitch must change as well.

In fact, however, listeners continue to match the pitch of the filtered complex to 200 Hz. We can remove more low-frequency components of the complex, and still a listener will match the pitch to 200 Hz. This auditory phenomenon, commonly referred to as the **case of the missing fundamental**, has been reported for harmonically related multiple pure tone complexes where the fundamental, or lowest frequency, is removed from the complex, resulting in no noticeable change in pitch. The explanation is that the components of both the original and filtered stimulus are harmonically related because each pure tone component is separated by 200 Hz. In other words, each pure tone component in both of the complexes is an integral multiple of the fundamental frequency of the complex (200 Hz), or a **harmonic**. Clearly, a place theory of pitch perception is not supported by this kind of empirical evidence.

In another example of pitch perception of a complex sound, we present the waveform shown in Figure 10-13a to a listener. This waveform consists of a

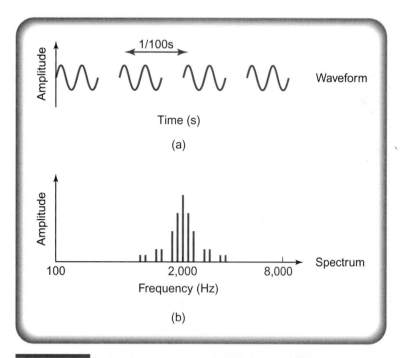

FIGURE 10-13 Schematic Illustrating Periodicity Pitch: A 2,000-Hz pure tone is periodically interrupted 100 times a second. The waveform (a) and the spectrum (b) of this stimulus are shown.

2,000-Hz pure tone that is interrupted 100 times per second. In other words, every 0.01 s, the 2,000-Hz pure tone turns on for a few cycles and then shuts off. Interrupting the pure tone 100 times per second significantly alters the spectrum of the 2,000-Hz tone, which is illustrated in Figure 10-13b. Most of the energy in the spectrum centers around 2,000 Hz, the frequency of the interrupted pure tone, but there is some energy spread into frequency regions higher and lower than 2,000 Hz. Because of the periodic temporal changes made to the pure tone, we do not see a single line spectrum.

We ask the listener to this complex stimulus to estimate its pitch. Place theory would predict that the subject would select a 2,000-Hz tone because this is the frequency of the interrupted tone and, more importantly, the maximum spectral energy of this stimulus is at 2,000 Hz. Maximum spectral energy corresponds to the place along the length of the basilar membrane responding with maximum displacement in the traveling wave response. Using this particular signal, that should correspond to the place along the basilar membrane corresponding to a center frequency of 2,000 Hz. When we perform a pitch experiment like this, however, we find that the listener matches the pitch of the stimulus to the interruption rate (100 times each second) rather than to the frequency of the pure tone (2,000 Hz). Pitch perception of interrupted pure tones is called **periodicity pitch** and cannot be explained by a simple place theory because the spectrum of the periodic complex stimulus usually has no spectral energy at the frequency corresponding to the assigned pitch.

Clearly we have two examples of our pitch perception to complex sounds that can't be explained using a place theory. However, would volley theory predict a different pitch estimate? Let's consider the case of periodicity pitch.

Figure 10-14a illustrates the complex waveform of an interrupted pure tone. Figure 10-14b shows the combined temporal pattern of neurological activity from this interrupted pure tone across the basilar membrane. According to volley theory, each time the interrupted pure tone is turned on, the combined neurological response involving the entire length of the basilar membrane will demonstrate bursts of neurological activity. The place where the activity occurs—the center frequencies of the critical bands—is not important in determining the pitch of the stimulus. What is important is the rate of neurological activity. Because the rate of neurological activity is locked to the temporal pattern of when the pure tone is on, the frequency of the pitch assigned will be the same as the interruption rate of the complex waveform. The place where the neurological activity occurs makes no difference to the pitch perceived. In fact, if we change the frequency of the interrupted pure tone, the pitch of the stimulus remains at the interruption rate, as long as that hasn't changed. Changing the frequency of the interrupted tone causes a change in the place where the activity occurs, but, according to volley theory, this isn't important to the frequency assigned to the stimulus pitch. Likewise, if we keep the frequency of the interrupted tone constant but change the rate of interruption, the pitch changes as well to follow the temporal characteristics of the stimulus.

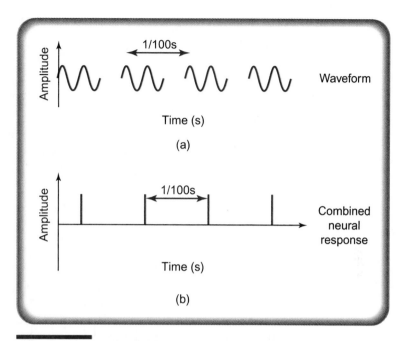

FIGURE 10-14 Explanation of Periodicity Pitch Using a Volley Theory of Pitch Perception: The waveform of an interrupted pure tone is shown, compared to the temporal pattern of overall neurological activity from the auditory nerve.

How does a volley theory of pitch perception account for the case of the missing fundamental? In the multitone complexes shown in Figure 10-12, the frequency separation between the pure tone components was 200 Hz. The overall temporal pattern of neurological activity provides bursts of activity corresponding to a rate equal to 200 Hz. So, even if the number of components making up the multitone complex is reduced, the overall neurological activity continues to show a temporal pattern corresponding to 200 Hz, the frequency of the assigned pitch. As we selectively remove more low-frequency pure tone components from the stimulus, the place on the basilar membrane corresponding to neurological activity changes, but not the overall temporal pattern of activity. Therefore, the pitch of the stimulus remains unchanged.

A MODERN-DAY THEORY OF PITCH PERCEPTION

Current theories of pitch perception include both a place and volley mechanism of pitch estimation. Figure 10-15 illustrates a current model of pitch perception by Moore (2003). An auditory stimulus moves serially through five levels of the model.

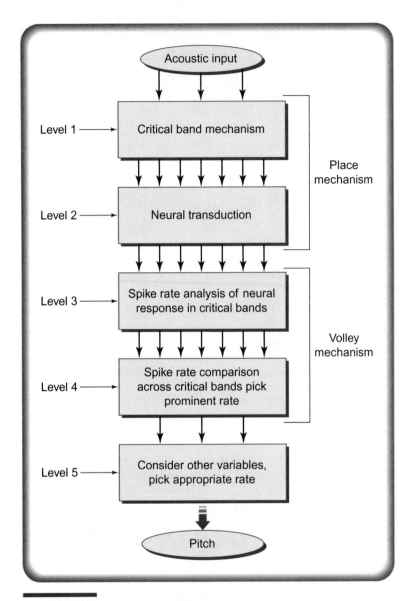

FIGURE 10-15 A Modern-Day Theory of Pitch. (Moore, 2003.)

- The first level is the critical band mechanism, which sifts the spectral energy of an incoming sound into the various critical bands with center frequencies equal to the spectral frequencies present in the signal.

- When filled with enough energy, the critical bands generate neurological activity. Critical bands that are empty or that contain less than a critical amount of energy remain quiet, in terms of their neurological activity.

These first two levels in Moore's model essentially represent the contribution of a place mechanism of pitch perception. The next three levels of the model represent a volley, or rate, mechanism to estimate pitch.

- In level 3, after the stimulus is sorted in terms of the critical bands, the rate of neurological activity is analyzed and coded across all the critical bands generating a response.

- In the fourth level, it is determined whether a consistent temporal pattern to the neurological activity of the responding critical bands exists.

- If a similar rate of neurological activity is found across several critical bands along the length of the cochlea, the last level in the model (level 5) evaluates this rate in light of the memory and attention characteristics of the listener, presentation characteristics of the stimulus, the context of the stimulus, and other listening and listener variables. This last level in the model makes the final decision regarding the frequency of the pitch assigned.

While this explanation of Moore's pitch perception model is oversimplified, the important point is the inclusion of both a place theory analysis and a rate theory analysis inherent in modern-day theories.

■ CHAPTER SUMMARY

We have covered several important concepts related to our perception of pitch. After reading and studying this chapter, you should be able to do the following:

- Provide a definition for the psychological perception of pitch.

- Describe the relationship between sound frequency and pitch.

- Compare and contrast the two primary ways hearing scientists obtain pitch estimates from listeners: direct and indirect procedures. Explain how these procedures are similar and in what important ways are they different. Provide an example of an experimental paradigm to illustrate each procedure.

- Define the direct unit of pitch, the mel.

- Compare and contrast the importance of stimulus intensity on pitch for soft versus very loud sounds.

- Provide a definition for the place theory of pitch perception and clearly explain the rationale behind the theory.

- Provide a definition for the volley, or rate, theory of pitch perception and clearly explain its rational.

- Compare and contrast the place and volley theories of pitch perception.

- Explain how the place theory of pitch perception adequately models our ability to judge frequency differences between pure tones.

- Explain how the place theory of pitch perception adequately models the change in pitch we perceive of a pure tone in the presence of a narrow band of noise.

- Define the case of the missing fundamental. Explain how the place theory of pitch perception cannot account for this phenomenon and how the volley theory can.

- Define periodicity pitch. Explain how the place theory of pitch perception cannot account for and how the volley theory can.

- Provide an illustration of a modern-day theory of pitch perception. Define the components, or levels, of processing in this theory and explain what kind of processing occurs at each level.

■ REFERENCES

Beck, J. and W. A. Shaw, "Single Estimates of Pitch Magnitude." *Journal of the Acoustical Society of America* 35 (1963): 1722–1724.

Cohen, A. "Further Investigation of the Effects of Intensity upon the Pitch of Pure Tones." *Journal of the Acoustical Society of America* 33 (1961): 1363–1376.

Fletcher, H. and W. A. Munson."Loudness, Its Definition, Measurement, and Calculation." *Journal of the Acoustical Society of America* 5 (1933): 82–108.

Moore, B. C. J. In *An Introduction to the Psychology of Hearing,* 5th ed. San Diego, CA: Academic Press, 2003.

Sivian, L. J. and S. D. White. "On Minumum Audible Sound Fields." *Journal of the Acoustical Society of America* 4 (1933): 288–321.

Small, A. M. "Psychoacoustics." In *Normal Aspects of Speech, Hearing, and Language,* 1st ed., edited by F. D. Minifie, T. J. Hixon, and F. Willians, 343–420. Upper Saddle Rive, NJ: Prentice Hall, 1973.

Stevens, J. C. and E. Tulving. "Estimations of Loudness by a Group of Untrained Observers." *American Journal of Psychology* 70 (1957): 600–605.

Stevens, J. C. and J. Volkmann. "The Relation of Pitch to Frequency: A Revised Scale." *American Journal of Psychology* 53 (1940): 329–353.

Stevens, J. C., J. Volkmann, and E. B. Newman. "A Scale for the Measurement of the Psychological Magnitude of Pitch." *Journal of the Acoustical Society of America* 8 (1937): 185–190.

Snow, W. B. "Changes of Pitch with Loudness at Low Frequencies." *Journal of the Acoustical Society of America* 8 (1936): 14–19.

Tobias, J. V. "Periodicity Pitch." In *Foundations of Modern Auditory Theory,* Vol. I, edited by J. V. Tobias, 1–54. New York: Academic Press, 1970.

SECTION FOUR

DURATION

■ DURATION AS AN IMPORTANT STIMULUS VARIABLE TO AUDITORY PERCEPTION

In this section, we turn our attention to a final stimulus parameter that significantly affects our perceptions to sounds: stimulus duration, which, quite simply, is the length of time a sound is present to a listener. We discover that a sound's duration does not affect our auditory perceptions unless the sound is relatively short. The influence of stimulus duration is rather limited compared to the influence of stimulus intensity and frequency. This is not to say, however, that stimulus duration has no effect on our auditory perceptions or that it is not important. When stimulus duration is brief enough to alter our auditory perceptions, its influence is significant.

We explore how stimulus duration influences a number of perceptual judgments we can make regarding the sounds we hear. We begin in Chapter 11 by examining several experimental studies looking at the effect of stimulus duration on sensitivity to pure tones and noise. We discover that the effect of duration on detection depends on a critical duration. For sounds shorter than this critical duration, sensitivity depends on the duration of the sound, and evidence suggests that the ear can trade the effects of duration and intensity to maintain audibility. We also examine experimental evidence concerning how duration influences our perceptions of the loudness of a sound.

Chapter 11 continues with a discussion of the effects that stimulus duration has on our auditory discrimination abilities. We explore experiments designed to measure the limits of our ability to discriminate temporal differences between sounds and compare our discrimination ability across frequency, intensity, and duration. The chapter ends with a discussion of the influence of stimulus duration on our discrimination ability of other acoustic parameters of a sound.

Chapter 12 discusses the processes of two important auditory phenomena in which stimulus duration plays a major role. Long-term poststimulatory auditory fatigue is a condition in which exposure to relatively intense sounds for relatively long periods of time brings about a temporary change in auditory sensitivity. We discover how the effects of long-term poststimulatory auditory fatigue are measured in a laboratory setting and the important conditions of the experimental setting that influence the magnitude of the effect.

A discussion of a second auditory phenomenon, loudness adaptation, concludes Chapter 11. We learn what loudness adaptation is and what typical listening environments bring about this effect. We study an experimental procedure that hearing scientists have used to illustrate and measure loudness adaptation. Finally, we explore the major differences between long-term poststimulatory auditory fatigue and loudness adaptation, in terms of the stimulus parameters usually required to bring about each phenomenon, the kinds of changes to auditory perception brought about by each phenomenon, and the characteristics of the ear's recovery from each phenomenon.

11

STIMULUS DURATION AND ITS ROLE IN AUDIBILITY, LOUDNESS, AND DISCRIMINATION

LEARNING OBJECTIVES

The important concepts you will learn in this chapter are:

- The influence of stimulus duration on absolute thresholds of detection for noise and pure tones.

- How stimulus duration and intensity are represented by the ear and how these stimulus variables are traded for relatively short durations of a sound.

- The definition, process, and characteristics of temporal integration.

- The influence of stimulus duration on loudness perception.

- The characteristics of normal human differential thresholds for duration.

- A comparison of the limits of our ability to discriminate the major acoustic variables of a sound.

- The influence of stimulus duration on our discrimination ability of other acoustic parameters of a sound.

KEY TERMS

Critical Duration

Discrimination Threshold for Duration (ΔT)

Method of Constant Stimuli

Stimulus Duration

Temporal Integration

Time-Intensity Trade

■ OVERVIEW

Having explored some important concepts related to the significance of stimulus intensity and stimulus frequency on our auditory perceptions, we now turn to a final acoustic parameter that may significantly influence our auditory perceptions. **Stimulus duration** is the length of time a sound is presented to a listener. In this chapter, we discover how stimulus duration affects our auditory perceptions to sounds. We address such questions as:

- Do the temporal characteristics of a sound influence its detectability and our psychological perception of loudness?
- How well are we able to discriminate temporal differences between sounds?
- Can the duration of a sound influence our discrimination abilities for other acoustic parameters of a signal, namely frequency and intensity?

We address these issues in this chapter.

■ STIMULUS DURATION AND AUDIBILITY

Small, Brandt, and Cox (1962) studied the effect of signal duration on the detectability of a wideband noise. Twelve normal-hearing listeners were presented with a number of wideband noise stimuli ranging in duration from less than 1 ms through 3 s (3,000 ms). Absolute thresholds, in decibels sound pressure level (dB SPL), were obtained for the signals throughout the durational range. Their results are presented in Figure 11-1, which demonstrates a two-part function

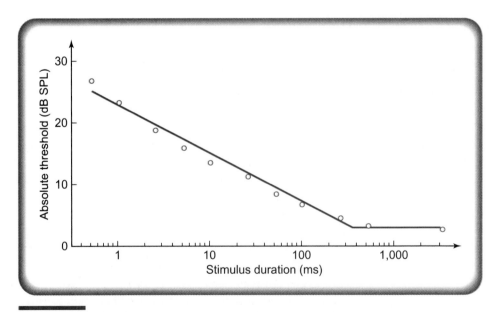

FIGURE 11-1 The Effect of Stimulus Duration on Detection Thresholds of a Wideband Noise. (After Small, Brandt, and Cox, 1962, from Small, 1973.)

relating absolute threshold as a function of stimulus duration. For signals shorter than 300 ms or so, absolute thresholds are linearly related to duration: As duration decreases, threshold increases. In other words, absolute threshold is *inversely* related to duration. As the duration of the signal shortens, audibility decreases; therefore the intensity of the stimulus must increase to keep it detectable. For signals characterized by durations greater than 300 ms, however, increasing duration further has no effect on threshold. In other words, a 500-ms wideband noise has the same absolute threshold as a 1,000-ms noise. For sounds characterized by relatively short durations, audibility apparently depends on the duration of the sound. For sounds characterized by relatively long durations, audibility is independent of duration. The critical point, where duration no longer influences audibility, seems to be about 300 ms, at least for wideband noise stimuli. Hearing scientists refer to 300 ms as the **critical duration**.

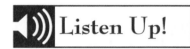 Listen Up!

AUDIBILITY OF SHORT-DURATION PURE TONES

Studies similar in design to Small, Brandt, and Cox have been reported using pure tones. The results from these studies suggest the same effect for critical duration as for wideband noise signals. However, these pure tone results differ from those reported using noise stimuli in terms of the magnitude of the critical duration. Some studies show that the critical duration changes with the frequency of the pure tone stimulus (Plomp and Bouman, 1959; Watson and Gengel, 1968); others have found critical duration independent of frequency (Olson and Carhart, 1966). Regardless of these discrepancies, it appears that, for very short tonal signals, audibility depends on the duration of the signal. Thresholds to longer tones, however, are independent of duration.

These results suggest that, within a critical range of duration, the ear is able to trade the effects of duration and intensity to keep the signal audible. In other words, stimulus audibility can increase or decrease by changing *either* intensity or duration. A change to either of these stimulus parameters produces the same change in threshold. Sounds of longer duration don't demonstrate this behavior, in that increasing the duration further doesn't make the signal more or less audible.

The ability of the auditory system to trade the effects of time and intensity for signals characterized by short durations is what hearing scientists refer to as **temporal integration**. The term "integration" is used in the mathematical sense as a way of combining the effects of time and intensity to bring about a change in audibility.

Figure 11-2 illustrates the concept of temporal integration for short signal durations.

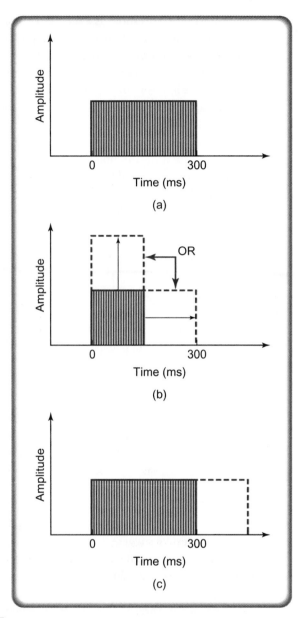

FIGURE 11-2 Temporal Integration: (a) An audible signal 300 ms in duration. The shaded area equals a critical amount of stimulus energy generated within the ear. (b) The same signal but with a duration reduced to 150 ms. To regain the amount of critical energy required to be audible, the signal must either increase in amplitude or increase in duration. (c) The condition where the signal has the same amplitude as in the top panel, but the duration exceeds 300 ms. The additional area of the rectangle is not integrated with the total energy of the original stimulus; so the absolute threshold to the signal does not change.

- Figure 11-2a is a schematic representation of the energy of a 300-ms wide band noise at threshold. The energy that this signal generates can be thought of as a *mathematical product* of the amplitude of the stimulus and the amount of time it's present in the auditory system. You can think of the shaded rectangle as the area that, when it achieves a critical magnitude, the stimulus is perceived.

- Figure 11-2b illustrates what happens when the signal is presented again, at the same amplitude but at a duration of 150 ms. Obviously, the area of the new pattern is only one-half of what it was previously. Because the shaded area is a reflection of the overall energy representation of the stimulus and because now the area is less than the critical magnitude suggested in (a), the stimulus is no longer audible. To make the stimulus audible again, we need to increase the area of the pattern. We can do this in one of two ways: (1) Keep the sound's duration at 150 ms but increase the amplitude; (2) keep the amplitude the same but increase the duration. It doesn't matter which way you choose to increase the overall energy representation of the stimulus, the consequence is the same: The tone becomes audible. This symbiotic relationship between stimulus intensity and stimulus duration, to maintain audibility, is referred to as the **time-intensity trade**.

- Figure 11-2c shows the effect of increasing the duration of a sound *beyond* the critical duration of 300 ms. The audible 300-ms stimulus energy is represented as the product of stimulus amplitude and time it is presented to the system (the shaded rectangle). The additional area brought about by increasing the duration of the stimulus isn't integrated into the original rectangle. Therefore, the overall energy representation of the stimulus doesn't change, which coincides with empirical evidence suggesting no change in detection threshold with duration, once the critical duration is achieved.

These studies of the effect of duration on thresholds of audibility seem to suggest that the duration of a stimulus does play a role in determining the absolute threshold to the stimulus, but only within limits. The effect of duration on audibility depends on relative duration:

- If the sound is characterized by a duration greater than a critical amount, duration does not affect the relative audibility of the sound.

- If the sound's duration is less than some critical amount, duration is important in determining threshold.

As the duration of very short sounds is decreased, detection threshold increases, suggesting that audibility suffers. Further, for very short duration sounds, intensity and duration are apparently represented or coded in the same way by the ear, such that a change in audibility caused by a change in one can be offset by a change in the other.

The ability of the ear to trade the effects of duration with the effects of intensity to keep a stimulus audible doesn't seem to hold for sounds with relatively long durations.

STIMULUS DURATION AND LOUDNESS PERCEPTION

In addition to demonstrating temporal integration of bursts of wideband noise, Small, Brandt, and Cox also investigated the influence of signal duration on loudness perception. Using a traditional loudness balance procedure, the investigators paired bursts of wideband noise, varying in duration between 0.4 ms and 500 ms, with a wideband noise of longer duration. The listeners adjusted the intensity of the shorter noise burst so that it had a loudness equal to the longer noise. Equal loudness contours were generated for low-, mid-, and high-intensity levels of the longer noise. In each case, Small, Brandt, and Cox discovered that, for very short durations of noise, the subjects adjusted the intensity of the second, shorter, noise to *higher* intensity levels, compared to the intensity of the standard sound.

The researchers interpreted these results as suggesting that, for very short durations of a wideband noise, *loudness decreases as duration decreases*. They also discovered that, once a critical duration was reached for the shorter variable stimulus, further increases in duration did not bring about a change in the listeners' loudness perception. The critical durations where loudness appears to be influenced by duration depended on the intensity level of the standard stimulus. The critical duration became longer as the intensity of the standard decreased. The important point, however, is that the effect of stimulus duration on loudness is demonstrated only for sounds characterized by extremely short duration, less than 10–50 ms, depending on the presentation level of the noise. We can conclude that, for the most part, stimulus duration *does not play a significant role* in determining our perception of loudness.

STIMULUS DURATION AND DISCRIMINATION

We have seen that stimulus duration plays a role in determining the audibility of sounds, at least in some situations, and that it may alter our loudness perceptions, but perhaps in more limited conditions. Now we turn our attention to the relative influence that stimulus duration may have on our ability to discriminate sounds.

DIFFERENTIAL THRESHOLDS FOR DURATION

The smallest difference in duration that can exist between two sounds to judge them as being different is our **discrimination threshold for duration (ΔT)**.

Small and Campbell (1962) reported the results of a study exploring this threshold. Using the **method of constant stimuli**, they asked 47 normal-hearing young adults to make judgments regarding pairs of wideband noise bursts. The

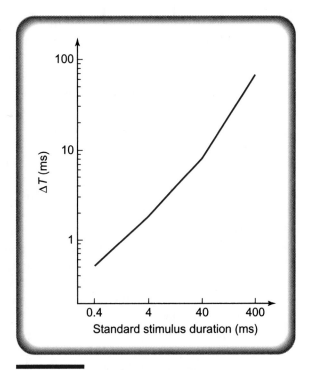

FIGURE 11-3 Difference Limen for Duration as a Function of Duration for a Wideband Noise. (After Small and Campbell, 1962, from Small, 1973.)

first noise of the pair, the standard, was presented at an intensity equivalent to 50 phons and ranged in duration from 0.4 ms through 400 ms. The second noise of the pair, the variable, was presented at durations that were considerably shorter or considerably longer than that of the standard. The subjects listened to the standard stimulus, followed by the variable stimulus, and judged whether the second sound was longer or shorter than the first. Discrimination thresholds for duration were calculated, in the usual way, for each duration of the standard stimulus.

Figure 11-3 plots average discrimination threshold, ΔT, as a function of the four durations of the standard stimulus. As the duration of the standard stimulus increases, so does the magnitude of ΔT. Given how small values of discrimination threshold are usually associated with relatively good resolution and larger values of discrimination threshold with relatively poor resolution, Small and Campbell were surprised by their results. They expected to see evidence of relatively poor temporal resolution for short durations of the standard and better temporal resolution ability as the duration of the standard increased. Their results, however, suggested the opposite trend.

Why would temporal discrimination be relatively good for very short bursts of noise and become progressively poorer as the duration of the noise grew longer? The answer, they concluded, has to do with the spectral changes that occur when the duration of a sound, in this case a wideband noise, is made very short. Recall the symbiotic relationship between the spectrum of a sound and its waveform: If the spectrum changes, the waveform changes, and vice versa. Because a wideband noise is characterized by random amplitude changes over time, for very short temporal samples of the wideband noise, the waveform can appear very different from one sample to the next. As the duration of the wideband noise increases, the waveforms of two samples become more alike because the random amplitude changes are averaged over a longer period of time. Small and Campbell hypothesized that the relatively small ΔT values they recorded from their listeners at very short noise durations were due to the subjects' detecting waveform differences between the standard stimulus and the variable stimulus, rather than differences in duration. As the durations of the standard and variable stimuli increased, the differences in the waveforms lessened; so the listeners had to rely on the perception of temporal difference to judge the noise pairs as being different.

Therefore, the suggestion that our temporal discrimination ability is relatively good at short durations and becomes poorer at longer stimulus durations is likely false. The ear is probably using two different cues to judge differences between the noise pairs: spectral differences at short durations and temporal differences at longer durations. This finding highlights a basic problem in measuring discrimination ability for very short duration signals. It is sometimes very difficult to tease apart our discrimination abilities across the temporal domain from our abilities across the frequency domain.

Comparison of Discrimination Ability for Important Acoustic Parameters

We can now compare the relative effects of stimulus intensity, frequency, and duration on our discrimination ability. Across a large range of values, our differential sensitivity for intensity wins overall, closely followed by frequency. In some listening situations, however, our ability to discriminate small changes in frequency is better than our ability to detect small changes in intensity. Therefore, with regard to our differential sensitivity for important acoustic properties of sound, we can reasonably conclude that:

- Our ears are well suited and quite capable of making distinctions between sounds based on their differences across intensity, frequency, and duration.
- Our ability to discriminate sounds depends on the type of discrimination (intensity, frequency, or duration) and on listening conditions.

- Under *ideal circumstances,* we can discriminate frequency changes as small as 1 or 2 parts in 1,000, intensity changes of 1 or 2 parts in 100, and temporal changes 1 or 2 part in 10 (Small, 1973).

- The auditory system has a tremendous discrimination ability for very small differences in a sound's frequency and intensity characteristics. Comparatively, the ear's ability to detect changes within the temporal domain is very crude.

THE EFFECT OF STIMULUS DURATION ON OTHER DIFFERENTIAL THRESHOLDS

Hearing scientists have also investigated whether stimulus duration affects our discrimination ability regarding other major stimulus parameters. In other words, is our overall ability to discriminate differences in intensity and in frequency the same whether the stimulus duration is very short or relatively long? Two investigations help us address this question.

The Effect of Stimulus Duration on Differential Thresholds of Intensity

In 1944, Miller and Garner reported results from a series of investigations designed to test whether the method by which sounds are presented to a listener affects the characteristics of the psychometric function and the magnitude of the discrimination threshold calculated from the function. To test their hypothesis, they measured discrimination thresholds for intensity using a 500-Hz pure tone of moderate audibility. The duration of the standard pure tone was varied. Although the intent of their investigation was not to measure the effect of stimulus duration on intensity discrimination, the results offer some insight into its effect.

Figure 11-4 presents a view of their results that suits our discussion. Intensity discrimination threshold is plotted as a function of the duration of the standard 500-Hz tone. The data suggest that intensity discrimination threshold remains relatively constant as the stimulus duration increases from about 250 ms through 750 ms. For signal durations shorter than 250 ms, however, ΔI increases with further reductions in standard stimulus duration. This result suggests that, for signals characterized by durations shorter than about 250 ms, our discrimination ability for intensity becomes poorer; we need larger differences between the intensity of the standard and variable stimulus to reliably judge them as being different. However, further increases in stimulus duration beyond 250 ms do not seem to affect intensity discrimination ability. Apparently, then, stimulus duration does not affect our ability to discriminate differences in stimulus intensity unless the duration of the stimuli is very short.

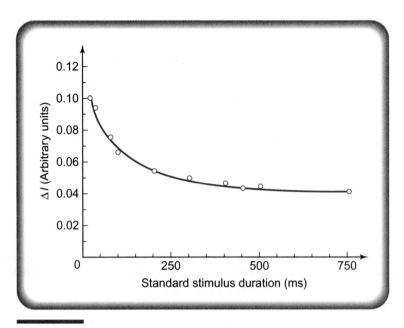

FIGURE 11-4 Difference Limen for Intensity as a Function of Duration for a 500-Hz Pure Tone. (After Miller and Garner, 1944, from Small, 1973.)

The Effect of Stimulus Duration on Differential Thresholds of Frequency

The duration of a stimulus may also influence our ability to discriminate frequency differences between sounds in certain limited conditions. Almost 50 years ago, Chih-an and Chistovitch (1960) measured frequency discrimination thresholds in normal-hearing listeners for a variety of short-duration pure tones.

Figure 11-5 presents their findings. It plots frequency difference limens, ΔF, as a function of signal duration for a 1,000-Hz pure tone. Again we see evidence of poorer frequency discrimination thresholds for stimulus durations less than about 300 ms. For durations shorter than this critical duration, ΔF increases as duration decreases. Likewise, for tone durations longer than 300 ms, ΔF is independent of duration; the threshold remains constant as duration increases further. Therefore, as was the case with intensity discrimination, duration does not appear to be a major stimulus variable affecting our ability to discriminate frequency differences between sounds, except those of relatively short durations. This is not to say that stimulus duration plays no role in our ability to discriminate sounds across other acoustic parameters, such as intensity and frequency. In addition, we certainly do encounter everyday sounds of very short durations. Speech, for example, is characterized by many sounds that are known for their brief durations. However, the

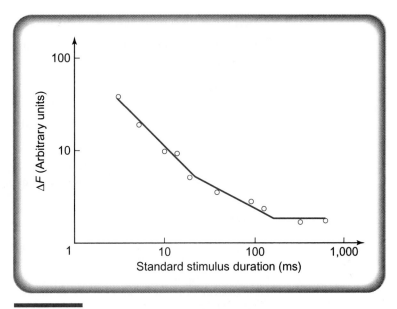

FIGURE 11-5 **Difference Limen for Frequency as a Function of Duration for a 1,000-Hz Pure Tone. (After Chih-an and Chistovitch,1960, from Small, 1973.)**

effect of duration on our ability to detect and discriminate sounds is limited to only these short sounds.

The effect of stimulus duration on our auditory perceptions continues to be an area of interest for hearing scientists and speech scientists alike. This chapter has presented the elementary concepts relating to stimulus duration and to its role in affecting audibility and simple auditory discrimination. By no means a complete picture of our current understanding of the importance of stimulus duration, the chapter merely provides a framework for ongoing study.

■ CHAPTER SUMMARY

We have covered several important concepts related to stimulus duration. After reading and studying this chapter, you should be able to do the following:

- Describe the relationship between stimulus duration and detection thresholds for wideband noise and pure tones.

- Define the concept of a critical duration as it relates to the audibility of a sound.

- Define temporal integration and show how this auditory process relates to the ear's ability to trade off the effects of time and intensity to maintain the audibility of a stimulus.

- Describe the effect of stimulus duration on our loudness perceptions.

- Describe our discrimination ability for duration as a function of wideband noise duration.

- Identify and explain the problems inherent in measuring differential thresholds for duration for very short duration sounds.

- Compare and contrast our relative discrimination ability for frequency, intensity, and duration.

- Describe how stimulus duration affects our ability to discriminate differences in stimulus intensity and in stimulus frequency.

REFERENCES

Chih-an, L., and L. A. Chistovitch. "Frequency Difference Limens as a Function of Tonal Duration." *Soviet Physics-Acoustics* 6 (1960): 75–79.

Miller, G. A. and W. R. Garner. "Effect of Random Presentation on the Psychometric Function: Implications for a Quantal Theory of Discrimination." *American Journal of Psychology* 57 (1944): 451–467.

Olson, W. O. and R. Carhart. "Integration of Acoustic Power at Threshold by Normal Hearers." *Journal of the Acoustical Society of America* 40 (1966): 591–599.

Plomp, R. and M. A. Bouman. "Relation Between Hearing Threshold and Duration for Tone Pulses." *Journal of the Acoustical Society of America* 31 (1959): 749–758.

Small, A. M. "Psychoacoustics." In *Normal Aspects of Speech, Hearing, and Language*, 1st ed., edited by F. D. Minifie, T. J. Hixon, and F. Williams, 343–420. Upper Saddle River, NJ: Prentice Hall, 1973.

Small, A. M., J. F. Brandt, and P. G. Cox. "Loudness as a Function of Signal Duration." *Journal of the Acoustical Society of America* 34 (1962): 513–514.

Small, A. M. and R. A. Campbell. "Temporal Differential Sensitivity for Auditory Stimuli." *American Journal of Psychology* 75 (1962): 401–410.

Watson, C. S. and R. W. Gengel. "Time-Intensity Trading Relations as a Function of Signal Frequency." 76th Meeting of the Acoustical Society of America, paper A7, 1968.

12

AUDITORY FATIGUE AND ADAPTATION

LEARNING OBJECTIVES

The important concepts you will learn in this chapter are:

- The importance of signal duration as it relates to the phenomena of long-term poststimulatory auditory fatigue and loudness adaptation, as well as typical listening situations that illustrate each.
- An example of an experimental paradigm used to measure the effects of long-term poststimulatory auditory fatigue and the measurement unit used to calculate the magnitude of long-term poststimulatory auditory fatigue for a particular listening condition.
- The experimental parameters affecting the relative amount of long-term poststimulatory auditory fatigue measured for a listening condition.
- An example of an experimental paradigm used to measure the effects of loudness adaptation.
- Important experimental characteristics of loudness adaptation.
- Loudness adaptation as a useful auditory process.
- The salient differences between long-term poststimulatory auditory fatigue and loudness adaptation.

KEY TERMS

Adapting Ear
Bounce
Comparison Ear
Control Condition
Experimental Condition
Fatiguer
Fatiguing Stimulus
Long-Term Poststimulatory Auditory Fatigue

Loudness Adaptation
Perstimulatory Phase
Poststimulatory Phase
Prestimulatory Phase
Recovery Interval
Simultaneous Dichotic Loudness Balance
Temporary Threshold Shift (TTS)

■ OVERVIEW

At a really loud concert of a particular sort, the music is presented at an intensity that we can feel just as much as hear. After a few hours of listening, when we leave the concert, we notice that our audibility to the sounds around us is impaired. Speech and other sounds just don't seem as detectable as they were before the concert. Our sensitivity to sounds is decreased, or made poorer, by the acoustic environment we have subjected ourselves to. Given time to recover, however, we notice our auditory sensitivity improving, and we experience a return to normal levels of detection.

In this example of a fairly common listening condition, we are experiencing the effects of **long-term poststimulatory auditory fatigue**. The degree of perceptual impairment is very much related to the duration of this kind of auditory exposure. Of course, the overall intensity level of the listening environment plays a significant role as well. For instance, this phenomenon hardly ever occurs if you sit for an hour or so at an orchestral concert, where the sound levels are usually much lower.

Here is another commonplace situation. In class, you happen to have picked a seat where something is buzzing: perhaps the lights above you, the heating/cooling system, or the projection device. Whatever is the source, it's producing a constant auditory stimulus that is not particularly loud, but definitely noticeable. Though the sound might be annoying at first, as you listen to the professor's lecture (because it is so fascinating), you notice sometime later that the buzzing doesn't sound as loud as before. You can still hear it, but the loudness has decreased to a point that it's not as annoying. This is an example **loudness adaptation**, which is the process of getting used to, or adapting to, the presence of a sound that doesn't significantly change its acoustic properties over time.

With both long-term poststimulatory auditory fatigue and loudness adaptation, the temporal characteristics of the signal play a major role in determining how certain aspects of our auditory perceptions change. In this chapter, we explore the experimental conditions and the auditory consequences related to auditory fatigue and adaptation that are relevant to many everyday listening conditions.

■ LONG-TERM POSTSTIMULATORY AUDITORY FATIGUE

Simply stated, long-term poststimulatory fatigue occurs when a high-intensity auditory stimulus is presented to the ear over a relatively long period of time. We experience the effects of exposure to this stimulus as a change in the ear's sensitivity after the stimulus stops.

Figure 12-1 illustrates the experimental paradigm used to measure auditory fatigue. The detection threshold of a sound, the signal, is measured in two conditions. Figure 12-1a shows the **control condition**. The absolute threshold of the

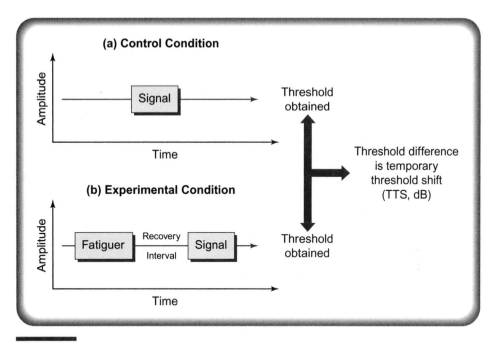

FIGURE 12-1 An Experimental Paradigm to Measure the Effects of Long-Term Poststimulatory Fatigue.

signal is obtained. Figure 12-1b shows the **experimental condition**, in which the subject is presented with a relatively long-duration, high-intensity sound. We call this sound the **fatiguing stimulus**, or the **fatiguer**.

The fatiguing stimulus is then shut off, and the ear is allowed to rest, or recover, for a period of time, a silent interval called the **recovery interval** and measured in units of time. Recovery intervals can last for any length of time. After the recovery interval has passed, the experimenter presents the signal, and absolute threshold is obtained. The thresholds to the signal for the two conditions are compared, and the difference between the thresholds (expressed in decibels) is defined as the **temporary threshold shift (TTS)**.

Figure 12-2 illustrates the experimental paradigm of a hypothetical study measuring the long-term fatiguing effects of a wideband noise on a 1,000-Hz pure tone signal. In the control condition, a simple detection threshold is obtained for the 1,000-Hz pure tone—let's say, 10 dB SPL. For the experimental condition, the listener is exposed for 30 min to a wideband noise fatiguer presented at 100 dB SL. After 30 min, the wideband noise is shut off, the ear is allowed to rest for 2 min, and the 1,000-Hz signal is presented. The threshold for the signal in this condition is measured to be 28 dB SPL. Finding the difference between the two thresholds (28 – 10 dB SPL), the experimenter records the TTS as 18 dB.

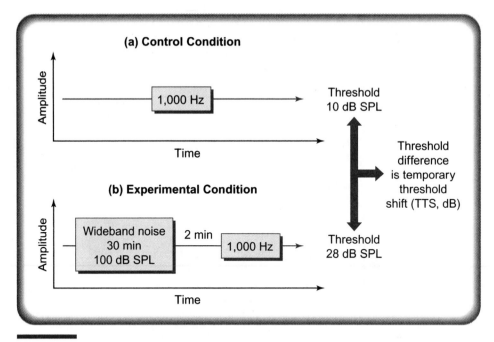

FIGURE 12-2 Hypothetical Experiment Measuring the Effects of Long-Term Poststimulatory Fatigue: A 30-min exposure to a wideband noise fatiguer is presented
at 100 dB SPL on a 1,000-Hz pure tone signal.

INTERPRETING THE MAGNITUDE OF TTS

The magnitude of TTS indicates the *degree* of influence the fatiguer has on signal
detection. The greater the magnitude of TTS that is measured after exposure to a
fatiguer, the more influence the fatiguing stimulus has on the detectability of the
signal. Likewise, the smaller the magnitude of TTS measured by the experimenter,
the less influence the fatiguer has on the audibility of the signal. An experimental condition that yields 0 dB TTS means that exposure to the fatiguing stimulus
resulted in no change to the detection threshold of the signal.

Suppose the experimenter changes the parameters of the experimental condition in Figure 12-2. The experimenter could do this by changing either the intensity
of the fatiguing stimulus or the duration of exposure to the fatiguing stimulus, or by
allowing the listener to recover longer before obtaining the threshold to the signal.
Whatever the made, we would expect a change in the amount of TTS recorded.

Assume that the experimenter decreases the exposure time to the fatiguing
stimulus to 10 min, while keeping the other parameters of the experimental condition the same. Suppose the new TTS obtained is 10 dB. By decreasing the duration
of exposure to the fatiguer, the amount of TTS observed decreases from 18 to 10 dB.
The influence of the fatiguer in the first experiment was greater than its influence in
the second experiment when the exposure time is less. Put another way, the change

in sensitivity to the 1,000-Hz pure tone brought about by the exposure to the wide-band noise fatiguer is greater in the first experiment, compared to the second.

The values of TTS may range from 0 dB up through any positive value, but TTS can never be a negative value. In other words, exposure to a fatiguing stimulus can never improve sensitivity to a signal. Exposure to a fatiguer has either no effect on sensitivity or causes sensitivity to become poorer.

EXPERIMENTAL PARAMETERS AFFECTING THE AMOUNT OF TEMPORARY THRESHOLD SHIFT

Experimental evidence suggests that the amount of TTS measured from a listener using the experimental paradigm illustrated in Figure 12-1 varies, depending on the acoustic characteristics of the fatiguing stimulus and on the duration of the recovery interval. There is empirical evidence related to each of these parameters in terms of their influence on TTS magnitude.

The Effect of the Recovery Interval on TTS

Figure 12-3 presents a particularly illustrative example of the effect of recovery interval duration on the magnitude of TTS (Hirsh and Bilger, 1955). Five listeners were exposed to a 1,000-Hz pure tone fatiguer for 4 min. The intensity of the

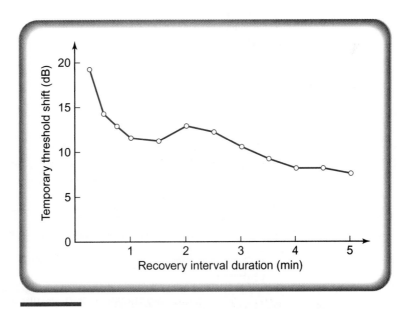

FIGURE 12-3 Effect of Recovery Interval Duration on Temporary Threshold Shift: Recovery is after exposure to a 1,000-Hz pure tone fatiguing stimulus at 100 dB SL for 4 min (1,400-Hz pure tone signal). (Data from Hirsh and Bilger, 1955.)

fatiguing tone was 100 dB SL, and the signal was a 1,400-Hz pure tone. Plotted is the average amount of TTS, in dB, for the five subjects as a function of recovery time.

The time course of recovery is interesting. An initial rapid decline in TTS is followed by an increase in TTS within the first 2 min of recovery. After 2 min, TTS declines slowly with time in a linear fashion. This was described by Hirsh and Bilger as a multiphasic recovery function, and it is characteristic of recovery functions after exposure to moderate- to high-intensity levels of the fatiguing stimulus. This multiphasic function had been reported by other scientists before Hirsh and Bilger; in fact Hirsh and Ward (1952) named the recovery function between 0 min and 2 min the **bounce**. Beyond recovery durations of 2 min, past the bounce, recovery occurs gradually and linearly over time. This appears to be a common characteristic of threshold recovery, regardless of the type of fatiguer and signal used or of the intensity of the fatiguing stimulus and exposure time (Dixon, Glorig, and Sklar; 1959a; Dixon, Glorig, and Sklar; 1959b).

The Effect of Fatiguer Intensity on TTS

The intensity of the fatiguing stimulus plays a major role in the amount of TTS recorded. Figure 12-4 shows data from Hirsh and Bilger illustrating this

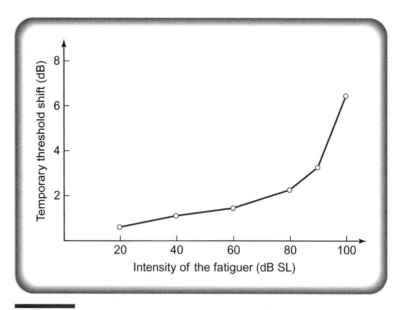

FIGURE 12-4 Effect of the Intensity of the Fatiguing Stimulus on Temporary Threshold Shift: Results after exposure to a 1,000-Hz pure tone fatiguing stimulus at a number of different intensity levels of the fatiguer and exposure times (1,400-Hz pure tone signal). (Data from Hirsh and Bilger, 1955.)

relationship. Plotted are averaged TTS values for five listeners after 3 min of recovery as a function of the intensity of the fatiguing stimulus. Again, the fatiguing stimulus was a 1,000-Hz pure tone, and the signal was a 1,400-Hz tone. The function is averaged over a number of exposure durations to the fatiguer, which ranged from 10 s through 4 min. Figure 12-4 shows that the amount of TTS is *directly related* to the overall intensity of the fatiguing stimulus. The increase in TTS magnitude seems especially significant for the highest levels of fatiguer intensities investigated.

The Effect of Exposure Duration on TTS

Ward, Glorig, and Sklar (1959a) were interested in the effects of narrow noise bands on TTS. Figure 12-5 illustrates a portion of their findings. Average TTS values from 26 ears are plotted as a function of exposure duration to a 105-dB SLP narrow band of noise. Notice that the scale of the abscissa is logarithmic. The bandwidth of the noise was 1,200 Hz, centered at 1,800 Hz, and the signal was a 4,000-Hz pure tone. Clearly, the amount of TTS is directly related to the duration of exposure, implying that the longer a listener is exposed to a fatiguing stimulus, the greater the effect the fatiguer has on sensitivity.

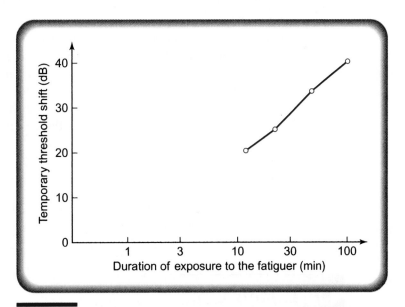

FIGURE 12-5 Effect of the Duration of Exposure to the Fatiguing Stimulus on Temporary Threshold Shift: Results after exposure to a narrow band of noise at 105 dB SPL (4,000-Hz pure tone signal). (Data are from Ward, Glorig, and Sklar, 1959a.)

SUMMARY REMARKS REGARDING LONG-TERM POSTSTIMULATORY AUDITORY FATIGUE

The effects of exposure to a high-intensity stimulus for relatively long periods of time are measured in terms of a temporary disruption of our sensitivity to sounds. The level of disruption depends, in predictable ways, on the acoustic properties of the fatiguing stimulus and on the characteristics of the listening environment. Major variables affecting the temporary changes we observe and their overall influence can be summarized as follows and *in general*:

- The longer we allow the ear to recover from the effects of a fatiguing stimulus, the less disruption we observe to our sensitivity. The time course of recovery is complex in the early stages, but after 2 min, TTS and recovery duration are inversely and linearly related.

- The more intense the fatiguer is, the more disruption we observe to auditory sensitivity. The relationship between TTS and the intensity of the fatiguing stimulus is direct, but it doesn't appear to be linear. In other words, exposure to sounds with very high intensities appears significantly more disruptive to our sensitivity than sounds with relatively moderate intensities.

- The longer we are exposed to a fatiguing stimulus, the greater the change is to our sensitivity. The relationship between TTS and the duration of exposure is direct.

- The effects of sounds bringing about measurable amounts of TTS are *temporary*. Eventually, given enough time to recover, the ear returns to its normal sensitivity levels. This is not to say, however, that *repeated* exposure to sounds that bring about TTS are harmless. Hearing scientists and audiologists alike have long suspected a relationship between temporary changes to sensitivity and permanent hearing loss. The exact nature of this relationship is not clear and continues to be investigated.

◼ LOUDNESS ADAPTATION

Loudness adaptation is the ear's way of getting used to the ongoing presence of a sound. Evidence of adaptation is apparent in all our senses, especially for sight and smell.

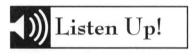

ADAPTATION IN ANOTHER SENSORY SYSTEM

Imagine that you are preparing an apple pie from scratch. When the pie is put into the oven to bake, you are likely to be very aware of the aroma initially. The smell of the pie baking seems pronounced. After a while, however, you might notice that the aroma isn't as strong as it once was. You can still smell it, but its magnitude has diminished. However, as soon as your friends come into your kitchen, they are very aware of the pie in the oven. (I hope you have some vanilla ice cream to go with that pie!)

The ear is not much different from the nose. If we are presented with an auditory stimulus that doesn't change much over time, the loudness of the stimulus appears to diminish the longer we listen to it. Initially, the sound is noticeable and may even be annoying. After a period of time, we might still perceive the sound, but the loudness has lessened; its apparent loudness has waned. Again, the length of exposure to the stimulus has a major influence on adaptation.

MEASURING LOUDNESS ADAPTATION

Unfortunately for beginning students of hearing science, measuring loudness adaptation in the laboratory is not nearly as straightforward as measuring long-term poststimulatory auditory fatigue. Because adaptation in the auditory system brings about a change in the *loudness* of a stimulus, rather than a change in threshold, its measurement must include some method of loudness estimation.

In his investigation into loudness adaptation, Thwing (1955) used a loudness balance procedure, although one a bit more complicated than what we have seen previously. Thwing refers to his procedure as a **simultaneous dichotic loudness balance**, primarily because both ears are presented with stimuli at the same time.

Figure 12-6 illustrates Thwing's experimental paradigm, in which the stimuli are presented to each ear in three phases of the study. One ear of the listener is designated as the **adapting ear**, the ear that is presented with the stimulus bringing about adaptation. The other ear is termed the **comparison ear**, the ear that is providing the loudness balance.

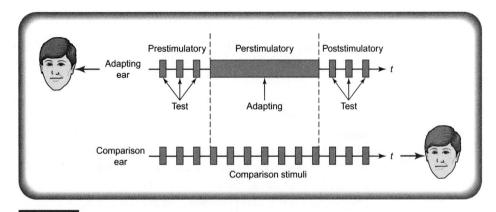

FIGURE 12-6 Experimental Paradigm Used by Thwing (1955) to Measure Loudness Adaptation. (After Thwing, 1955.)

- In the first phase of the experiment, the **prestimulatory phase**, the same signal is delivered to each ear. Notice that the sounds delivered to each ear are pulsed: 20 s on and 90 s off. In the prestimulatory phase, the listener is asked to adjust the intensity of the stimulus delivered to the *comparison ear* so that it is equally loud to the stimulus presented to the adapting ear. Once loudness is balanced between the two ears, the prestimulatory phase ends, and the perstimulatory phase begins.

- In the **perstimulatory phase**, the stimulus presented to the *adapting ear* becomes continuous. The comparison stimulus, on the other hand, continues to be pulsed. The subject's task in this phase of the experiment is to adjust the intensity continuously in the comparison ear to match the loudness in the adapting ear. The perstimulatory phase is generally much longer in duration than the prestimulatory phase.

- In the **poststimulatory phase**, the adapting stimulus is changed from a continuous sound back to a pulsing sound. The time course of the presentation of the adapting stimulus changes to its characteristics in the prestimulatory phase. The comparison signal continues to pulse and has not changed. The subject again is required to adjust the intensity of the comparison stimulus so that it is equally as loud as the stimulus in the adapting ear.

Thus, the listener is providing a real-time loudness balance to what is being perceived in the adapting ear. In addition, the loudness balance is performed before the adapting stimulus is presented (prestimulatory phase), during the presentation of the adapting stimulus (perstimulatory phase), and after the presentation of the adapting stimulus (poststimulatory phase). By noting how the intensity of the comparison stimulus changes before, during, and after the presentation of the adapting stimulus, Thwing was able to infer how loudness changed, over time, in the adapting ear.

IMPORTANT CHARACTERISTICS OF LOUDNESS ADAPTATION

Some of Thwing's (1955) results are illustrated in Figure 12-7. These data include conditions where both the adapting and comparison sounds were 1,000 Hz pure tones, but the intensity of the adapting tone was kept to 80 dB SPL throughout all the phases of the study. The figure plots the intensity of the comparison tone adjusted by the listeners during the three phases of the experiment to keep the loudness perceived between the two ears the same. In other words, we get an indication of the *time course* of the real-time loudness balance. As the intensity of the comparison tone is lowered, the loudness of the stimulus in the adapting ear is *decreasing*. Similarly, as the intensity of the comparison tone is made higher, the loudness of the stimulus in the adapting ear is *increasing*. An abbreviated schematic of the experimental paradigm is represented at the bottom of the figure.

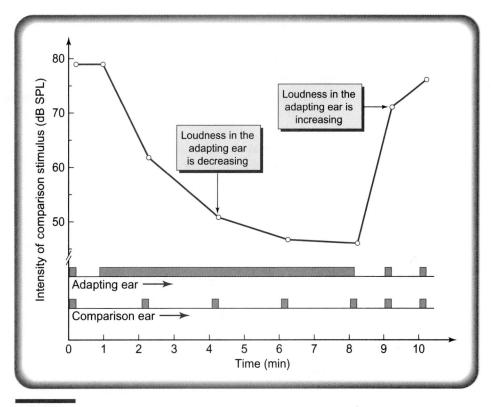

FIGURE 12-7 **Results from Thiwing's Loudness Adaptation Study. (After Thwing, 1955.)**

These results suggest several conclusions regarding the characteristics of loudness adaptation.

- First, we see that, during the prestimulatory phase of the experiment, the intensity of the comparison tone just about equals the intensity of the adapting tone for loudness to be the same in the two ears. This should not be surprising, because the tones delivered to both ears during this phase are identical.

- The perstimulatory phase of the experiment begins after 1 min and lasts for 7 min. During this time, we see that the listeners decrease the intensity of the comparison tone. During the first 3 min of the perstimulatory phase, the intensity of the comparison tone is decreased by about 30 dB from its original level, suggesting that the apparent loudness of the adapting tone is decreasing rapidly during this time.

- During the next 4 min, the intensity of the comparative stimulus decreases somewhat more modestly, suggesting that the loudness of the adapting tone continues to decline a bit further but levels off and doesn't change significantly after about 5 min of exposure.

- Finally, there is a dramatic increase in the intensity of the comparison tone between the end of the perstimulatory phase and the first minute of the poststimulatory phase of the experiment. This phenomenon suggests that, when the continuous adapting signal was changed abruptly to a pulsed tone, loudness increased markedly and rapidly. In fact, just after 2 min into the poststimulatory phase, the intensity of the comparison tone reaches a level of almost prestimulatory values.

The interpretation of these results suggests important characteristics regarding loudness adaptation.

- During the initial exposure to an adapting stimulus, the decrease in perceived loudness is steady and persistent. Maximum loudness reduction occurs during the first 3–4 minutes of exposure. After that, changes in loudness may continue to occur, but only modestly, suggesting that the overall change in loudness of the adapting stimulus eventually reaches a maximum value, after which longer exposure doesn't appear to reduce the loudness further. (During all this time, the adapting stimulus continues to be *audible*; only its perceived loudness has changed.)

- The recovery from loudness adaptation is rapid. Once the adapting stimulus has changed in terms of some acoustic aspect, its loudness increases markedly and very rapidly. The time course of recovery from the effects of adaptation is very, very short.

All these characteristics enable loudness adaptation to serve its purpose of allowing the ear to multitask. It allows the auditory system to put an unchanging and uninteresting stimulus on a back burner. The ear continuous to perceive the stimulus, but, as long as the sound remains unchanged, its relevance is reduced. In a way, the ear moves the stimulus off-line until something interesting happens. During adaptation, the ear becomes more alert to other auditory stimulation. In short, loudness adaptation is a way for the ear to acknowledge the presence of a sound but reduce its significance over time if nothing very interesting is changing in it. Although perception never disappears, the sound quickly moves to the forefront if its acoustic parameters change. The ear is then ready to devote its complete attention to the sound once again.

COMPARISON OF LONG-TERM POSTSTIMULATORY AUDITORY FATIGUE TO LOUDNESS ADAPTATION

Although the temporal factors of a sound are extremely important to its effects related both to long-term poststimulatory auditory fatigue and to loudness adaptation, these processes are distinct, both physiologically and psychologically. As you try to resolve the characteristics and effects of these processes in your own mind, consider these major differences:

- Auditory fatigue brings about a change in *sensitivity* in the ear, whereas adaptation brings about a change in *loudness*.

- Auditory fatigue concerns the effect that one stimulus has over the perception of another, but adaptation concerns the change in perception of a single stimulus over time.

- In general, the intensity of a stimulus causing auditory fatigue is greater than the intensity of a stimulus bringing about loudness adaptation.

- The time course of loudness adaptation, especially related to recovery, is much more rapid compared to auditory fatigue.

■ CHAPTER SUMMARY

We have covered several important concepts related to long-term poststimulatory auditory fatigue and loudness adaptation. After reading and studying this chapter, you should be able to do the following:

- Provide conceptual definitions and everyday listening examples of long-term poststimulatory auditory fatigue and loudness adaptation.

- Provide an example of an experimental paradigm used to measure the effect of long-term poststimulatory auditory fatigue and identify the important experimental parameters.

- Provide an example of calculating temporary threshold shift, the measurement unit of long-term poststimulatory auditory fatigue.

- Explain the consequences of increasing the magnitude of temporary threshold shift, as it relates to the effect of long-term poststimulatory auditory fatigue.

- Summarize the effects of recovery interval, fatiguing stimulus intensity, and fatiguing stimulus duration on long-term poststimulatory auditory fatigue.

- Provide an example of an experimental paradigm used to measure the effect of loudness adaptation and identify the important experimental parameters.

- Identify and describe the important auditory perceptual characteristics of loudness adaptation as they relate to loudness change.

- Explain the usefulness of loudness adaptation.

- Identify and describe four important ways that loudness adaptation and long-term poststimulatory auditory fatigue are different.

REFERENCES

Hirsh, I. J., and R. C. Bilger. "Auditory-Threshold Recovery After Exposures to Pure Tones." *Journal of the Acoustical Society of America* 27 (1955):1186–1194.

Thwing, E. J. "Spread of Per-stimulatory Fatigue of a Pure Tone to Neighboring Frequencies." *Journal of the Acoustical Society of America* 27 (1955): 741–748.

Ward, W. D., A. Glorig, and D. L. Sklar. "Temporary Threshold Shift from Octave-Band Noise: Applications to Damage Risk Criteria." *Journal of the Acoustical Society of America* 31 (1959a): 522–528.

Ward, W.D., A. Glorig, and D. L. Sklar. "Relation Between Recovery from Temporary Threshold Shift and Duration of Exposure." *Journal of the Acoustical Society of America* 31 (1959b): 600–602.

13

INTRODUCTION TO BINAURAL HEARING

■ OVERVIEW

Almost all the auditory perceptions and abilities discussed so far have been limited to monaural listening. Except for Sivian and White's (1933) minimum audible field condition for absolute threshold, monaural stimulus presentations have been a common condition in the experimental evidence that we have reviewed. The reason is, quite simply, that, when both ears are included in the listening condition, things get complicated. **Binaural listening** involves higher levels of the auditory system than monaural listening. The central auditory pathways are tapped into more heavily when listening with both ears than with one. Clearly, though, listening to sounds in everyday settings involves the use of both ears.

The complications associated with binaural conditions, however, don't mean we should ignore them entirely. This chapter presents a simple discussion of some of our fundamental auditory perceptions as binaural listeners. We also learn about some of the important acoustic cues that influence binaural perceptions. There is certainly a lot more to learn about binaural hearing than what is presented in this chapter; so, if you further your studies in hearing science, you will certainly investigate binaural hearing in greater depth. Chapter 13 is meant to highlight some of our simple binaural perceptions and offer rudimentary explanations for them.

■ LOCALIZATION

Localization is our ability to judge the direction and relative distance of a sound in a **sound field**. For example, when we hear the emergency siren of a moving police car or ambulance, we usually can sense the origin of the sound with respect to our position in space. We can tell whether the vehicle is in front of us, behind us, or off to one side. We sense its distance and its movement in space, again relative to our position.

All these auditory perceptions are related to our localization abilities and are very much a consequence of listening with two ears. To localize a sound in space, equal sensitivity between the two ears is essential. In fact, even hearing-impaired listeners maintain some localization ability, as long as the sensitivity of the two ears is about the same.

In this section we address the following questions:

- How does the auditory system perform localization?
- What acoustic cues does the auditory system use during localization?
- How are these cues employed?
- Are other kinds of auditory behaviors related to listening binaurally?

ACOUSTIC AND AUDITORY CUES INVOLVED IN LOCALIZATION

In general, the cues used for localizing a sound source in a sound field are related to the frequency of the sound and our discrimination ability regarding stimulus intensity and duration. How we make use of these cues depends, in large part, on the frequency of the sound source.

Higher-Frequency Sound Sources and Localization

Suppose a blindfolded listener is positioned in a sound field with a sound source some distance away off to the right side. The sound source is turned on and emits a high-frequency pure tone. We ask the listener, without the benefit of visual cues, to point in the direction of the sound. With a rather high degree of accuracy, the listener is able to consistently identify the direction of the sound source.

Figure 13-1 presents a schematic of this listening setting, and it should help us understand the acoustic cues from the high-frequency pure tone that the listener is using and, more importantly, how these cues are used. The listener is positioned in a sound field with the sound source to the right side. Because the sound wave emitted by the source is a high-frequency pure tone, the **wavelength** of the disturbance is relatively short. Recall that the wavelength (the distance from one complete cycle of oscillation to the next) is *inversely related* to frequency. Because of the relative proportion between the wavelength size and the size of the head, when the disturbance strikes the head, a shadow is cast, much like a shadow our body might

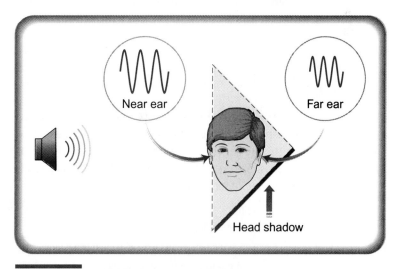

FIGURE 13-1 Illustration of the Important Acoustic Cues Used in Localizing High-Frequency Sounds.

cause by blocking light. The shadow, called **head shadow**, falls on the ear farther away from the sound source, and it is a consequence of the physical interaction of a short wavelength sound disturbance striking the relatively large head.

The primary effect of head shadow is a difference in the amplitude of the sound reaching the two ears. The ear closer to the source, the **near ear**, perceives the amplitude of the sound at a *higher intensity* than the ear farther from the source, the **far ear**. In other words, the physical intensity of the sound is greater in one ear than in the other. Depending on the frequency of the source, the intensity difference between the two ears can be as much as 20 dB (Feddersen, Sandel, Teas, and Jeffress, 1957), especially if the source is directly perpendicular to the near ear.

The intensity difference of the signal arriving at each ear is represented as a difference in the magnitude of the waveform, as illustrated in Figure 13-1. (The frequency of the sine wave in each ear is the same; there is no phase difference between the tones.) The waveform of the high-frequency pure tone generated in the near ear is larger than the one generated in the far ear. This is a direct consequence of the intensity difference of the signal as it enters each ear. Hearing scientists believe that the central auditory system compares the excitation patterns in the two ears to make judgments as to which ear is closer to the source. The ear with the higher internal representation of intensity—the ear closer to the source—is receiving the higher stimulus intensity. Recall that our ability to judge intensity differences between sounds is very good over a rather large range of stimulus intensities, on the order of 1–2 dB. Because the auditory system is very sensitive to small differences in intensity between the two ears, it can easily determine which ear is closer to the sound source.

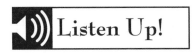

Listen Up!

THE MAGNITUDE OF THE HEAD SHADOW

The magnitude of the head shadow depends on the frequency of the sound source and on the position of the source relative to the listener. Head shadow is the greatest when the frequency of the source is high (5,000–10,000 Hz) and the source is directly perpendicular (90°) to one ear or the other.

- If the frequency of the sound source is lowered, the magnitude of the head shadow effect decreases.

- If the sound source changes from a 90° orientation with the head to directly in front of the listener (0°) or directly behind it (180°), the magnitude of head shadow decreases substantially (Feddersen, Sandel, Teas, and Jeffress, 1957).

The intensity differences between the two ears, used as an aid to localization, are referred to as either **interaural intensity differences** or **interaural level differences**. Because of our exquisite differential sensitivity for intensity, an interaural intensity difference detected by the auditory system between the two ears is a very powerful cue to determining our relative position to a sound source in a sound field, most prominently for higher-frequency pure tones.

Lower-Frequency Sound Sources and Localization

As the frequency of a sound source moves lower, the magnitude of the head shadow effect decreases. The auditory system must therefore make use of a different cue to determine the location of low-frequency signals in a sound field. Figure 13-2 illustrates the consequences of lower-frequency sounds reaching a listener in a sound field. The listener is situated, as in Figure 13-1, with a sound source directly off to the right side. The frequency of the pure tone is low, and, as a consequence, the wavelength of the disturbance is relatively long. Recall that, as the frequency of a pure tone decreases, the wavelength increases proportionately. When this sound wave strikes the head, it *bends* around the head, rather than casting a shadow. As a result, the intensity of the signal reaching each ear is about the same; so interaural intensity differences in this condition are minimal. (In the figure, the two sine waves are of equal amplitude.) What is different between the ears is the *arrival time* of the stimulus. The bending of the disturbance around the head to reach the far ear

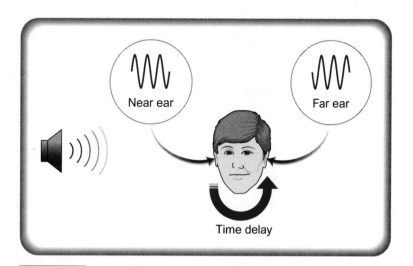

FIGURE 13-2 Illustration of the Important Acoustic Cues Used in Localizing Low-Frequency Sounds.

causes a brief delay in the arrival of the disturbance to the far ear. The near ear receives the signal first, followed by the far ear. Due to our differential sensitivity regarding temporal aspects of a stimulus, the auditory system is sensitive to the time-of-arrival differences.

Delaying the arrival of a tonal stimulus to one ear compared to the other is manifested in terms of a difference in the *phase* of the pure tone stimulus between the two ears. This effect is also illustrated in Figure 13-2. The waveform representation in the far ear is 180° out-of-phase with the waveform in the near ear. Because the pure tone arrives first at the near ear, the internal phase representation in that ear will be ahead of, or lead the far ear. The internal phase representation of the disturbance in the far ear is lagging that in the near ear, due to the delay in the time of arrival. Scientists believe that the central auditory system compares the phase representation generated in each ear and decides that the representation leading in phase is closer to the source—the ear that received the stimulus first. The ear with the internal phase representation lagging in phase is the far ear, which received the disturbance later in time. The phase differences between the two ears, used as an aid to localization and referred to as **interaural phase differences**, are the greatest for low-frequency pure tones perpendicular (90°) to one ear or the other.

- As the frequency of the sound source increases, the time-of-arrival differences between the ears decrease, as well as the differences in phase.

- As the sound source moves from a 90° orientation with the head to directly in front of the listener (0°) or directly behind it (180°), interaural phase differences decrease (Feddersen, Sandel, Teas, and Jeffress, 1957).

In summary, the acoustic and auditory cues that the auditory system uses for localization depend in large part on the frequency of the sound source.

- For low-frequency sounds, the system primarily relies on interaural phase differences between the two ears.

- For high-frequency sounds, it primarily relies on interaural intensity differences.

The idea that the auditory system uses two different cues for localization, depending on the relative frequency of the sound source, is sometimes referred to as the **duplex theory**. Interaural *phase* difference cues are a direct result of time-of-arrival differences between the ears. Interaural *intensity* difference cues are a direct result of the head's shadow causing a difference in the intensity of the sound reaching the two ears. Our differential sensitivity to stimulus intensity and stimulus duration allows us to discriminate the differences in the internal representation of the sound source between the two ears, thereby helping us to decide which ear is closer to the source.

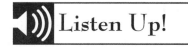 Listen Up!

LOCALIZATION CUES

The cues used for localization depend, in large part, on the frequency of the disturbance. At which frequency does the auditory system stop using interaural phase differences and start using interaural intensity differences as the dominant cue? In a series of experiments involving the localization of pure tones, Sandel, Teas, Feddersen, and Jeffress (1955) concluded that localization of tones below about 1,500 Hz is determined largely by interaural time differences. For frequencies above 1,500 Hz, differences of intensity at the two ears appears be the dominant factor.

OTHER AUDITORY PERCEPTIONS AS A CONSEQUENCE OF INTERAURAL PHASE AND INTERAURAL INTENSITY DIFFERENCES

Several other interesting auditory perceptions are related to binaural listening brought about by interaural phase and intensity differences between two sounds. These perceptions have to do with what I call the "laboratory version" of localization. Recall that localization occurs when a sound is presented in a sound field to a listener and both ears perceive the sound, that is, they are unoccluded. The binaural perceptions in this section occur when sounds are delivered simultaneously to both ears through headphones. Depending on the physical differences in the sounds, some interesting auditory perceptions can occur, particularly with two types of stimuli: pure tones and clicks.

Interaural Phase Differences and Binaural Beats

Suppose a listener is presented with two different pure tones that are delivered to each ear at the same time through headphones. The intensity of the pure tones is the same, but their frequencies differ by 5 Hz. For example, a 250-Hz pure tone is delivered to the right headphone, and a 255-Hz pure tone is delivered to the left headphone. The listener is asked to describe what she hears. You may be tempted to predict that the listener will report the perception of beats, and you would be partially right. The perception of primary beats is produced when two pure tones of slightly different frequencies are electronically mixed and presented, monaurally, to a listener (Chapter 6). The physical mixing of the two waveforms results in amplitude modulation, which creates our perception of a tone periodically changing loudness over time.

However, our listening condition is different: The two pure tones presented to the listener are not mixed electronically before being delivered to the listener. Rather, they are delivered dichotically, one stimulus to each ear. In **dichotic listening**, a different stimulus is presented to each ear simultaneously. In this case, the stimuli are two pure tones of slightly different frequencies. This is an important difference from the conditions that give rise to regular, primary beats because in this dichotic listening condition the two pure tones are "mixed" by the central auditory system, not by an electronic device. The interactions between the two pure tones in the dichotic presentation occur *neurologically* in the central auditory pathways, not before the tones are delivered to the peripheral auditory system.

Our listener would perceive a different kind of beat associated with something called **lateralization**, which is the perception that results from a dichotic presentation of two pure tones. A fused tonal auditory image appears to originate within the head that moves periodically from one ear to the other. The pure tone appears to move, inside the head, from the left ear up through the center of the forehead and continuing over to the right ear. As long as the pure tones continue playing, the perception of the tone moves back to the right ear in the same manner. The frequency with which the tone moves from one ear to the other equals the frequency difference between the two pure tones delivered to each headphone. The perception of this dichotic stimulus presentation is called **binaural beats**, to distinguish them from typical primary beats, which usually are brought about in a monaural presentation.

How does the auditory system represent and mix these stimuli, and, more importantly what auditory cues does the system use to give rise to our perception of binaural beats? The perception is due primarily to the auditory system's interpretation of the interaural phase differences between the two tones. Figure 13-3 illustrates how this works by plotting the waveforms of two pure tones, one delivered to each ear. The pure tones have the same amplitude and starting phase, but their frequencies are slightly different. When time begins, the phase of each pure tone delivered is the same. At this point in time, the auditory image is directly in the center of the head. As time continues, however, the ear presented with the higher-frequency pure tone (the left ear), begins to lead in phase because the period is a bit shorter compared to that of the other tone. Although in localization the stimulus that leads in phase indicates an earlier time of arrival, at this point the difference in the times of arrival between the two ears is not enough to move the image all the way over to the left ear. As the phase difference between the tones increases, however, the time-of-arrival cue gets bigger, and the auditory image moves closer to the leading (left) ear. Eventually, the temporal differences are great enough to push the auditory image all the way over to the left ear. As time continues, the phase differences between the tones continue in their cyclical pattern: One ear gradually moves toward leading in phase, then gradually moves toward lagging. The perception of the location of the image in the head directly follows the periodic phase changes between the two tones.

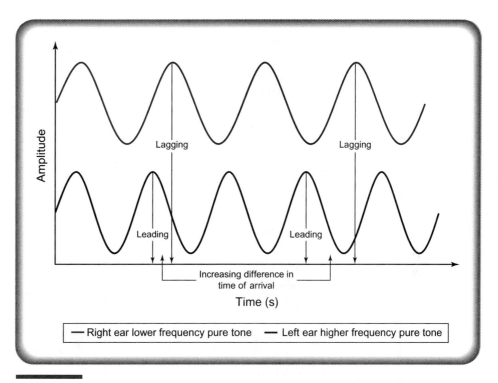

FIGURE 13-3 Important Temporal Characteristics of Two Waveforms Causing the Perception of Binaural Beats.

Interaural Intensity and Time-of-Arrival Differences and Lateralization

Another interesting binaural phenomenon we can create in a laboratory setting involves the use of click stimuli. **Clicks** are a type of impulsive sound characterized by extremely short durations and an infinite continuous spectrum. Though not readily encountered in everyday listening conditions, they are used widely in laboratory and clinical settings because they produce a robust physical response involving the entire length of the basilar membrane. Also, because of their short duration, they also provide a robust neural response from the auditory nerve.

In Figure 13-4a, a listener is presented with two click stimuli, one delivered to each ear, through headphones. The clicks have the same intensity and are delivered at exactly the same time to each ear. In other words, the interaural intensity difference is zero, as is the difference in time of arrival. The figure also shows the neurological responses for the right and left ears as a function of time. Notice that the robust neurological response arising from the clicks occurs at exactly the same time in each ear. If we ask the listener to describe the perception related to this

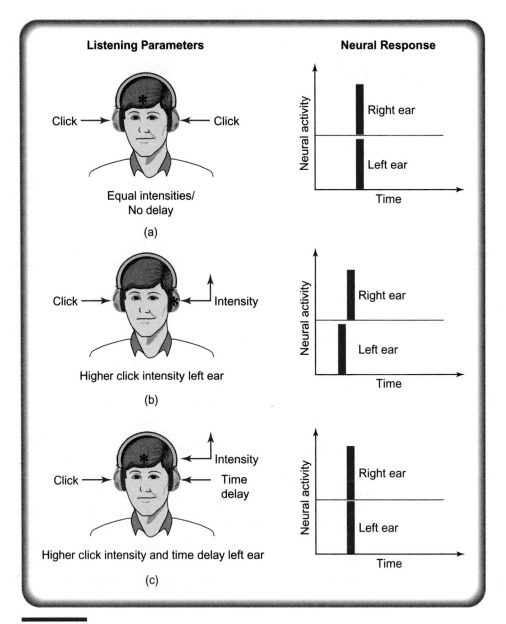

FIGURE 13-4 Illustration of the Important Acoustic and Neurological Cues Used in Lateralization of Click Stimuli.

presentation, the subject will describe a single fused auditory image at the center of the head (indicated by the asterisk). This response would appear to make sense because the magnitude and timing of the synchronous neurological burst of activity arising from the stimuli delivered to each ear are identical.

When we change the intensity of one click, while leaving the other click intensity unchanged, the resulting condition is shown in Figure 13-4b. Both clicks are delivered simultaneously to each ear (no time-of-arrival difference), but the intensity of the click presented to the left ear is higher than in the other ear. The listener, when asked to report perceptions, will indicate hearing a fused image in the left ear, the ear presented with the higher-intensity click. The image has lateralized from the center of the head (as was the perception when the intensity and time of arrival of the clicks were identical in each ear) to the left ear.

If we look at the neurological activity occurring in each ear as a function of time, we see why the image lateralizes to the left ear. The increase in the intensity of the click in the left ear has resulted in a *decrease in the latency* of the neural response in that ear. The higher stimulus intensity delivered to the left ear has caused the neurological burst of activity in the left ear to occur sooner. Therefore, the stimulus has arrived at the left ear first, and this is the ear to which the image lateralizes. Generally, as the intensity of a stimulus increases, the time it takes the neurological response in that ear to occur gets shorter. The time it takes the neurological response of the auditory pathways to become evident, after the onset of the stimulus, is the **latency period**. Increasing stimulus intensity brings about a reduction in the latency of the response.

Figure 13-4c shows one more change to the listening condition. The experimenter delays the presentation of the higher-intensity click in the left ear, and the click delivered to the right ear remains the same as in the previous two conditions. The small time delay in the left ear causes the auditory image to move toward the center of the head. If we were to increase the amount of delay in the left ear, ultimately the listener would report the image all the way over to the right ear. Thus, we can compensate for the lateralization effects of a more intense click presentation in one ear by delaying the presentation of the click, in time, in the same ear.

Using click stimuli presented dichotically, time of arrival and click intensity can be *traded* to move the sound image toward one ear or the other. This happens because both time of arrival and intensity differences between the two ears are represented neurologically by the auditory system as changes in response latency. Increasing click intensity reduces the latency of the neurological response, as does presenting the click sooner to the system. Both of these acoustic parameters of the clicks are represented by the auditory pathways in the same way.

■ BINAURAL MASKING LEVEL DIFFERENCES

A final binaural phenomenon with considerable clinical as well as scientific application is **binaural masking level differences**. This phenomenon is sometimes referred to as **release from masking** because it results in an improvement in auditory sensitivity when both ears are allowed to participate in a noisy listening condition.

The next time you're at a busy party, try listening to your friend with one ear occluded. Your understanding of what's being said will be more difficult. As soon as you unocclude your ear, however, speech understanding will most likely improve. By allowing two ears to have access to both the speech and the noise, the central auditory system is able to reduce the internal representation of the noise to make the speech more audible.

To measure binaural masking level differences, a noise stimulus, usually either wideband or narrow band, is delivered to each ear through headphones at a comfortable loudness level. The noise presented to each ear must originate from the same source and be split between the two ears. In addition to the noise, a pure tone is also delivered to each ear.

These listening conditions are illustrated in Figure 13-5. Masked thresholds to the pure tone delivered binaurally are obtained in two conditions. In Figure 13-5a, the pure tones are presented in-phase. In Figure 13-5b, the pure tones are presented 180° out-of-phase. The intensity of the pure tone required for threshold in each condition is recorded. The difference of the two masked thresholds, in decibels, is the magnitude of the binaural masking level difference.

Usually, depending on the frequency of the pure tone used, the threshold is lower when the tones are 180° out-of-phase between the two ears than when the tones are delivered in-phase. Just by inverting the phase between the two tones,

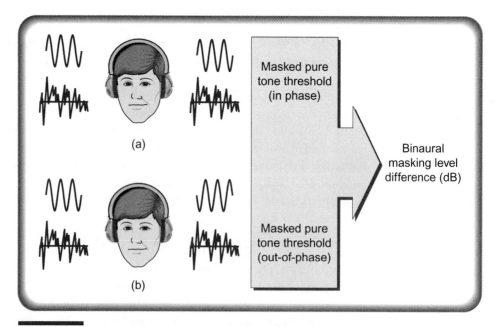

FIGURE 13-5 Measurement of Binaural Masking Level Difference.

sensitivity improves. This is the release from masking; the inverted phase of the pure tones reduces the effectiveness of the masker.

The magnitude of the masking level difference may vary across individual listeners and with the frequency of the pure tone presented to the listener. Generally, binaural masking level differences are large for low-frequency tones, and they decrease as the frequency of the tone increases. For instance, at 500 Hz, the masking level difference for most normal-hearing listeners is approximately 15 dB; at 1,500 Hz, however, the masking level difference drops to less than 5 dB (Moore, 2003).

Release from masking is not limited to tones. Masking level differences can occur for complex signals characterized by a significant amount of low-frequency spectral energy, such as speech. Normal masking level differences require normal central auditory functioning, at least at the level of the brainstem. Indeed, listeners having brainstem pathology generally show abnormally small masking level differences, which accounts for the usefulness of this binaural ability as a measure of auditory functioning in clinical applications.

The theories to explain release from masking are beyond the scope of this text. Suffice it to say, however, that, when both the internal representations of the signal and the noise from each ear meet in the central auditory system, the signal is separated somewhat from the noise. When this occurs, audibility is improved. Auditory pathology, especially involving the brainstem, inhibits the separation of speech from noise, resulting in limited improvement in audibility or none at all.

CHAPTER SUMMARY

We have covered several basic concepts related to binaural auditory ability. After reading and studying this chapter, you should be able to do the following:

- Define auditory localization and explain the necessary listening conditions and listener characteristics required for this auditory skill.

- Identify and explain the important acoustic cues for localizing high-frequency sounds.

- Define and describe the head shadow effect and its role in the localization of high-frequency sounds.

- Define interaural intensity differences and how the auditory system uses these differences in determining the direction of a sound.

- Identify and explain the important acoustic cues for localizing low-frequency sounds.

- Explain how differences in the time of arrival of a low-frequency sound between the two ears are represented in the auditory system as interaural phase differences. Describe how this difference is used as an aid to the localization of these sounds.

- Define binaural beats and explain the listening conditions that bring about this auditory perception.

- Explain the changes in our perception of click stimuli, presented dichotically, as the time of arrival is the same or different between the two ears and as the intensity is the same or different between the two ears.

- Describe how the time of arrival and the intensity of clicks are represented neurologically in the auditory system.

- Define release from masking.

- Describe how release from masking is measured in a laboratory or clinical setting as the binaural masking level difference.

- Identify and describe the important characteristics of the binaural masking level difference in terms of the frequency of the pure tones involved, the acoustic characteristics of the noise, and listener characteristics.

■ REFERENCES

Feddersen, W. E., T. T. Sandel, D. C. Teas, and L. A. Jeffress. "Localization of High-Frequency Tones." *Journal of the Acoustical Society of America* 29 (1957): 988–991.

Moore, Brian C. J. *An Introduction to the Psychology of Hearing*, 5th ed. New York: Academic Press, 2003.

Sandel, T. T., D. C. Teas, W. E. Feddersen, and L. A. Jeffress. "Localization of Sound From Single and Paired Sources." *Journal of the Acoustical Society of America*, 27 (1955): 2842–2852.

Sivian, L. J., and S. D. White. "On Minumum Audible Sound Fields." *Journal of the Acoustical Society of America* 4 (1933): 288–321.

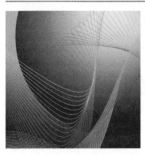

GLOSSARY

ΔF A way of referring to a discrimination threshold for stimulus frequency. *See also* Discrimination Threshold (ΔF).

ΔI A way of referring to a discrimination threshold for sound intensity. *See also* Discrimination Threshold for Intensity.

ΔS In experimental psychology, the smallest difference in a specified modality of sensory input that is detectable by a human observer.

ΔT A way of referring to a discrimination threshold for stimulus duration. *See also* Discrimination Threshold for Duration.

3-dB Down Point A reduction in the amplitude, usually expressed in power, that corresponds to one-half the original intensity of an input signal once passed through a filter. This typically corresponds to the upper and/or lower cutoff frequencies of a high-pass, low-pass, or band-pass filter.

A

Abscissa In an *x-y* plot, the name of the *x*-axis.

Absolute Threshold The magnitude of a stimulus necessary for the receiver to detect the presence of the stimulus 50 percent of the time.

Acceleration The rate of change in velocity or speed of an object over time.

Adapting Ear In a simultaneous dichotic loudness balance experimental design, the ear that is presented with the stimulus bringing about adaptation.

Amount of Masking The magnitude of the effect that a masker has on a signal. It is measured as the difference in the threshold of the signal in quiet to its masked threshold. The unit of amount of masking is the decibel (dB).

Amplitude A key characteristic of a sine wave. It is the magnitude or strength of the vibration.

Amplitude Modulation The amplitude change as a function of time of the resulting waveform when two pure tones of slightly different frequencies are combined.

Aperiodic A vibration that does not repeat itself over time.

Aperiodic Sounds A broad classification of types of sounds that do not repeat their waveforms regularly over time. Noise and transient sounds are two common kinds of aperiodic sounds.

Asymmetry of Masking The change in the masking pattern, or function, as masker intensity is increased, where the low-frequency side of the masking pattern becomes steeper while the high-frequency side of the masking pattern becomes shallower.

Atmospheric Pressure The pressure at any given point in the earth's atmosphere. In the waveform display of a pure tone, it represents equilibrium pressure.

Audibility The degree to which a sound can be detected.

Audiometric Zero A sound pressure level that corresponds to 0 dB in the HL reference. Audiologists expect normal-hearing listeners to be able to just detect the presence of any sound at levels equivalent to 0 dB HL. It corresponds to the lower limit of usable hearing, measured in the clinical setting. *See also* Hearing Level (dB HL).

Auditory Sensitivity The degree to which a listener is able to respond to external auditory stimuli.

B

Bandwidth In band-pass filtering, the width of the band of frequencies allowed to pass without significant reduction in amplitude.

Band-Pass Filter A frequency-selective attenuation device that diminishes the amplitude of input signal frequency components in the high and low frequencies. Input frequencies above and below the pass band are attenuated. Band-pass filters are made by passing an input signal through a high-pass and a low-pass filter in succession.

Bel (B) A unit of sound magnitude originally devised by engineers of Bell Telephone Laboratories to quantify the reduction in audio level over a 1-mile length of standard telephone cable. Ten decibels are equivalent to 1 bel (B).

Binaural Beats The perception that results from a dichotic presentation of two pure tones, differing slightly in frequency. The perception is that of a fused tonal image moving from one ear to the other within the head.

Binaural Listening Conditions characterized by listening with both ears.

Binaural Masking Level Differences Clinical and experimental measures of the improvement in auditory sensitivity that can occur under some binaural listening conditions.

Bounce A term coined by Hirsh and Ward (1952) to describe the changes in TTS values, as a function of time, for recovery intervals between 0 and 2 min.

C

Cancellation The resulting silence brought about by the addition of two sine waves with identical frequencies and amplitudes, but with a phase difference of 180°.

Case of the Missing Fundamental Auditory phenomenon in which the pitch of a complex periodic stimulus, consisting of harmonically related components, does not change as low-frequency components are removed from the stimulus. This phenomenon lends support to a volley, or rate, theory of pitch perception.

Center Frequency In a band-pass filter, the single frequency lying at the exact center of the bandwidth, or the range of frequencies allowed to pass through unattenuated.

Classical Theory/Place Theory of Pitch Perception An important theory of pitch perception formulated by Hermann von Helmholtz in 1863. The fundamental premise of this theory is that the pitch given to a signal ultimately depends on the place along the basilar membrane corresponding to the maximum displacement of the traveling wave response.

Clicks A type of impulsive sounds, characterized by extremely short durations and an infinite continuous spectrum.

Comparison Ear In a simultaneous dichotic loudness balance experimental design, the ear that is providing the loudness balance.

Completely Out-of-Phase The relationship of two sine waves that are 180° different in phase.

Complex Tones The result of the combination of two or more pure tones.

Complex Wave The result of the combination of two or more sine waves.

Comprehension In experimental psychology, the process by which meaning is extracted from a perceived stimulus. This is the fourth and final level in the hierarchy of auditory behavior.

Condensation During the propagation of a sound wave, regions of higher molecular density or pressure, compared to equilibrium.

Continuous Spectrum The type of spectrum typical of most aperiodic sounds. The frequency components making up a continuous spectrum are infinite and continuous throughout a broad range of frequencies.

Control Condition In the experimental paradigm used to measure long-term poststimulatory auditory fatigue, the condition where absolute threshold of the signal is obtained before exposure to the fatiguing stimulus.

Critical Band A model of frequency analysis of the peripheral auditory system, originally proposed by Fletcher (1940), suggesting that the basilar membrane can be thought of as containing a number of band-pass filters arranged serially according to center frequency. As we move down the length of the membrane, from base to apex, the center frequency of each of the band-pass filters decreases progressively, from high frequencies to low frequencies. Each ½ mm traveled represents a move to the next adjacent band-pass filter. Critical bands are sometimes referred to as internal auditory filters.

Critical Band Theory One of the cornerstones of psychoacoustic theory to explain how the peripheral auditory system represents, processes, and utilizes the stimulus parameter of frequency.

Critical Bandwidth The bandwidth of the critical bands, or internal auditory filters, hypothesized by Fletcher (1940).

Critical Duration An important time constant for the ear, which is approximately 300 ms. Generally, the ear processes sounds with durations of less than 300 ms differently, compared to sounds with durations longer than 300 ms.

Cutoff Frequency In terms of high-pass or low-pass filtering, the critical frequency at which spectral energy is either attenuated or allowed to pass through unchanged.

Cycle of Vibration One complete oscillation of an object vibrating periodically.

D

Decibel (dB) A logarithmic unit of measurement used to express the magnitude of a sound relative to a specified or implied reference level. Because it is the expression of a ratio between two quantities, it is a dimensionless unit. A decibel is one-tenth of a bel (B).

Density In physics, mass per unit volume.

Dependent Variable In the design of experiments, the variable representing the observed response from a subject brought about by controlled exposure to the independent variable. It is the data collected by the experimenter. In an *x-y* plot, the dependent variable is typically represented as the ordinate.

Detection In experimental psychology, the ability of an observer to perceive the presence of a stimulus and distinguish it from silence or its absence. This is the first and most basic level in the hierarchy of auditory behavior.

Dichotic Listening The listening condition characterized by presenting different sounds to each ear simultaneously though headphones.

Difference Limen (DL) In experimental psychology, the smallest difference in a specified modality of sensory input that is detectable by a human observer. *See also* Differential Thresholds of Sensitivity.

Differential Thresholds of Sensitivity A generic term for the smallest difference in a specified modality of sensory input that is detectable by a human observer. *See also* Difference Limen.

Direct Linear Relationship In an *x-y* plot, the relationship between the dependent and independent variables characterized by increasing levels of the dependent variable with increasing levels of the independent variable and a straight line.

Direct Magnitude Estimation (DME) A type of psychoacoustic experimental design in which listeners are required to provide ratio estimates of some psychological perception of a sound, based on their perception, to the same psychological perception for another sound whose physical characteristics are fixed by the experimenter.

Direct Magnitude Production (DMP) A type of psychoacoustic experimental design in which listeners are required to provide the physical characteristics of a sound, based on the ratio estimate of some psychological perception of a second sound. The ratio estimate is fixed by the experimenter.

Direct Procedures of Pitch Estimation Pitch estimation using either a direct magnitude estimation (DME) or a direct magnitude production (DMP) psychophysical procedure.

Discrimination In experimental psychology, the ability of an observer to judge or perceive a difference between two stimuli that differ in terms of some physical parameter. Discrimination is the second level in the hierarchy of auditory behavior.

Discrimination Ability for Intensity The ability of a listener to judge or perceive a difference between two sounds that differ in stimulus intensity. *See also* ΔI.

Discrimination Threshold (ΔF) In experimental psychology, the smallest difference in a specified modality of sensory input that is detectable by a human observer.

Discrimination Threshold for Duration The smallest possible difference between two sounds, in terms of duration, in order for a listener to judge them as being different. *See also* ΔT.

Displacement The magnitude of a vibration from equilibrium. It is similar to amplitude.

Duplex Theory The theory that the auditory system uses two different cues for localization, namely interaural intensity differences and interaural phase differences, depending on the relative frequency of the sound source.

E

Envelope of the Spectrum In the spectrum of an aperiodic sound, the envelope determined by connecting the amplitudes of the infinite frequency components throughout the spectral range of the sound. It provides an indication of the energy characteristics of the sound as a function of frequency.

Equal Loudness Contour Typically, the experimental evidence provided by Fletcher and Munson (1933). These are functions connecting the frequency and intensity characteristics of pure tones of equal loudness.

Equal Pitch Contours Typically, the experimental evidence provided by Snow (1936). These are functions connecting the frequency and intensity characteristics of pure tones of equal pitch.

Equilibrium The midpoint of vibration in an object vibrating with simple harmonic motion. It is the point where the net displacement of the vibration is zero.

Excitation Pattern A schematic representation of the total amount of neurological energy, or excitation, distributed across the length of the basilar membrane in response to a sound.

Experimental Condition In the experimental paradigm used to measure long-term poststimulatory auditory fatigue, the condition in which the subject is presented with a fatiguing stimulus. The fatiguing stimulus is then shut off, and the ear is allowed to rest. After recovery, the absolute threshold of the signal is obtained.

Experimental Paradigm In psychoacoustic experimental design, a schematic representation of the number, duration, frequency, or intensity of sounds presented to the subjects, as a function of time. The judgments the listener must provide regarding the stimuli may also be included in the figure.

Exponential Notation In mathematics, a way of writing numbers that accommodates values too large or too small to be conveniently written in standard decimal notation. Numbers are displayed as a decimal number between 1 and 10 followed by an integer power of 10.

F

Far Ear In a sound field listening condition, the ear farther from the sound source.

Fatiguer Another name for a fatiguing stimulus.

Fatiguing Stimulus A long-duration, high-intensity stimulus that results in long-term poststimulatory auditory fatigue.

Filter A frequency-selective attenuation device

Filter Skirt The attenuation characteristics of an output spectrum from a high-pass, low-pass, or band-pass filter, beyond the cutoff frequency.

Fourier Analysis The mathematical process of deconstructing complex vibrations to their constituent waves. It is the reverse of Fourier synthesis.

Fourier Synthesis The mathematical process of combining sine waves to produce more complex vibrations. It is the reverse of Fourier analysis.

Frequency The numerical expression of the number of cycles or oscillations per unit time, typically 1 s. It is a key characteristic of a sine wave, The unit of frequency is cycles/s (cps) or hertz (Hz). Frequency is inversely related to the period.

Frequency Difference Limen (DL) The smallest frequency separation that a listener can perceive between two sounds that differ in terms of stimulus frequency.

Frequency Discrimination Threshold The smallest frequency separation that a listener can perceive between two sounds that differ in terms of stimulus frequency. It is synonymous with frequency difference limen.

Frequency Selectivity The relative ability of the ear to perceive differences in stimulus frequency.

Function In an *x-y* plot, the relationship between the dependent variable and the independent variable.

G

Graph A diagram depicting the relationship between two or more variables used to visualize scientific data.

H

Harmonic For complex periodic tones consisting of harmonically related components, a component frequency of the signal that is an integer multiple of the fundamental frequency.

Head Shadow A consequence of the physical interaction of sound striking the head in a sound field listening condition. The consequence of this interaction is a reduction in the sound pressure level of the signal reaching the ear that is farther away from the source compared to the closer ear. This effect is most pronounced for higher-frequency tones.

Hearing Level (dB HL) A common reference for the decibel that is based on the typical sound pressure levels of sounds that normal-hearing, young adults need just to be able to detect their presence. This reference is primarily used in the clinical measurement of hearing.

Helium A colorless, odorless, tasteless, nontoxic element that is less dense than air.

Hertz (Hz) The accepted unit of frequency, named in honor of Heinrich Rudolf Hertz. The old unit of frequency, cycles/s (cps), was renamed in 1960 by the General Conference on Weights and Measures.

Higher Cutoff Frequency In band-pass filtering, the higher-frequency limit of the pass band. It is determined by the cutoff frequency of the low-pass filter of the filter series.

High-Pass Filter A frequency-selective attenuating device that diminishes the amplitude of low-frequency components of a signal and allows the high-frequency components to pass with full original amplitude.

I

Independent Variable In the design of experiments, the variable that the experimenter deliberately manipulates to invoke a change in the dependent variable. In an *x-y* plot, the independent variable is typically represented as the abscissa.

Indirect Method of Loudness Estimation A psychophysical design method of estimating loudness only at the point of loudness equality. The loudness unit of estimates derived in this fashion is the phon.

Indirect Procedures of Pitch Estimation A psychophysical design method of estimating pitch only at the point of equality.

Input Signal In filtering, the spectrum of a signal entering a filter.

Intensity One of two ways to represent physical sound magnitude used in the calculation of a decibel equivalent. The unit of sound intensity is watt/cm^2, where a watt is a unit of work or power.

Interaural Intensity Differences The intensity differences between the two ears in sound field listening conditions, primarily resulting from head shadow. This intensity cue is used as an aid to localizing higher-frequency tones.

Interaural Level Differences The intensity differences between the two ears in sound field listening conditions, primarily resulting from head shadow. This intensity cue is used as an aid in localizing higher-frequency tones. Synonymous with interaural intensity differences.

Interaural Phase Differences A consequence of time-of-arrival differences between the two ears in sound field listening conditions. The ears represent the difference between the times of arrival of the stimulus as a difference in the phase of the stimulus between the two ears and uses it as an aid to localizing lower-frequency tones.

Inverse Relationship A mathematical relationship in which one variable decreases as a second one increases.

J

Just Noticeable Difference (jnd) In experimental psychology, the smallest difference in a specified modality of sensory input that is detectable by a human observer. *See also* DL and Differential Thresholds of Sensitivity.

L

Latency Period Regarding the neurological behavior of single auditory neurons, the time it takes, after the onset of the stimulus, for the neurological response in the ear to become evident.

Lateralization The perception that results from a dichotic presentation of two pure tones.

Line Spectrum The type of spectrum typical of most periodic sounds. The spectrum is characterized by one or more finite pure tone frequencies, or lines, of measurable amplitude.

Linear Projection In simple harmonic motion, the one-dimensional representation of an object moving with uniform angular velocity.

Linear Scale A graphical representation in which each incremental change on one end of the scale is equal to the same incremental change on the other end of the scale.

Localization Our ability to judge the direction and relative distance of a sound in a sound field.

Logarithmic Scale A graphical representation based on an abstract mathematical unit that is defined as being proportional to the value of a logarithm function.

Longitudinal Wave Motion A type of wave motion in which the particles in the medium move in the same direction as the propagation of the disturbance. Sound waves exhibit this type of wave motion.

Long-Term Poststimulatory Auditory Fatigue A phenomenon that occurs when a high-intensity auditory stimulus is presented to the ear for a relatively long period of time. The effect of exposure to this stimulus is measured as a change in the ear's sensitivity after the stimulus has been turned off.

Loudness The perceptual quality of sound related to sound intensity but not solely determined by it.

Loudness Adaptation The apparent reduction in loudness perceived in response to a constant, fixed stimulus.

Loudness Balance Procedure An example of an indirect method of loudness estimation. In this procedure, a listener is required to adjust the intensity of a stimulus until its loudness is equal to that of another stimulus, whose physical parameters are fixed by the experimenter.

Loudness Summation The auditory perception of increasing loudness of a noise with increasing bandwidth of a noise of constant energy. This auditory phenomenon supports the existence of the critical bands.

Lower Cutoff Frequency In band-pass filtering, the lower-frequency limit of the pass band. It is determined by the cutoff frequency of the high-pass filter in the filter series.

Low-Pass Filter A frequency-selective attenuation device that diminishes the amplitude of the high-frequency components of a signal and that allows the low-frequency components to pass with full amplitude.

M

Masked Threshold The threshold of a signal in the presence of a masker whose acoustic parameters are fixed by the experimenter.

Masker In masking, the stimulus that may interfere with the detection of the signal.

Masking The process by which the simultaneous presence of one sound interferes with the detection of another.

Masking Function The graphical representation of the amount of masking as a function of signal frequency.

Maximum Peak Amplitude One way to express the amplitude of a sine wave. It represents the maximum number of amplitude units that the sine wave possesses in either the positive or negative direction, or the magnitude of the excursion from equilibrium.

Medium One of the three necessary components of a sound system. The medium consists of molecular particles that transmit the vibrations of the source to the receiver. The plural of medium is media.

Mel The unit of pitch resulting from a direct pitch-scaling procedure. One thousand mels is equivalent to the pitch of a 1,000-Hz pure tone presented with an intensity of 40 dB SL.

Method of Constant Stimuli One of several traditional psychophysical experimental procedures employed by hearing scientists. This classical psychophysical method is often used to estimate discrimination thresholds in listeners.

Minimum Audible Field (MAF) The threshold of audibility as a function of frequency for pure tones presented to normal-hearing listeners by a loudspeaker 1 m away.

Minimum Audible Pressure (MAP) The threshold of audibility as a function of frequency for pure tones presented monaurally to normal-hearing listeners through headphones.

Model A description or a theory to explain the empirical evidence of behavior.

Monaural Relating to, affecting, or designed for use with one ear.

N

Narrow-Band Noise Wideband noise that is filtered in such a way as to restrict the range of frequencies it covers.

Near Ear In a sound field listening condition, the ear closer to the sound source.

Noise One type of aperiodic sound. The waveform is characterized by random fluctuations of amplitude as a function of time.

O

Ordinal Scale A type of numbering system or scale in which the numbers representing the scale can be compared in terms of greater and lesser, as well as equality and inequality. Mathematical operations of addition and subtraction, however, are meaningless.

Ordinate In an x-y plot, the name of the y-axis.

Oscillation In terms of vibration, the mechanical movement of an object.

Output Signal In filtering, the spectrum of the signal coming out of a filter.

P

Parameter The independent variable not represented by the abscissa in a graph of an experiment with two independent variables.

Pascal (Pa) A unit of pressure equivalent to newton/m^2. The unit was renamed in 1971 in honor of Blaise Pascal, a French mathematician, physicist, and philosopher who lived in the seventeenth century.

Peak-to-Peak Amplitude One way to express the amplitude of a sine wave. It represents the overall amplitude of the sine wave, in both the positive and negative directions. Peak-to-peak amplitude takes into account the full magnitude of excursion around the equilibrium.

Period A key characteristic of a sine wave. It is the numerical expression of the time taken for the wave to complete one cycle, or oscillation. The unit of period is time, usually expressed in seconds. The period is inversely related to frequency.

Periodic A characteristic of vibrations that repeat their oscillations regularly as a function of time.

Periodic Sounds The broad classification of types of sounds that repeat their waveforms regularly over time.

Periodicity Pitch A phenomenon related to pitch estimates from listeners presented with interrupted pure tones. The pitch estimation is based on the interruption rate of the tone rather than the frequency of the interrupted tone. This phenomenon lends support to a volley, or rate, theory of pitch perception.

Perstimulatory Phase The second of three stages of a simultaneous dichotic loudness balance experimental paradigm.

Phase A key characteristic of a sine wave. It is related to the relative position of an object vibrating with simple harmonic motion at in a moment of time during its oscillation and how this position compares with other vibrating objects.

Phase Locking A characteristic of the neural activity of single auditory nerve fibers, where the time pattern of a fiber's neural activity is tied to the phase of the stimulating tone.

Phons Units of loudness estimation derived from an indirect method of loudness estimation. Phons reflect an ordinal numbering system or scale.

Pitch The perceptual quality of sound related to frequency, but not solely determined by stimulus frequency.

Pitch Matching An example of an indirect method of pitch estimation. In this procedure, a listener is required to adjust the frequency of a stimulus until its pitch is equal to that of another stimulus, whose physical parameters are fixed by the experimenter.

Pressure In physics, the force over an area applied on an object in a direction perpendicular to the surface.

Prestimulatory The first of three stages of a simultaneous dichotic loudness balance experimental paradigm.

Poststimulatory Phase The last of three stages of a simultaneous dichotic loudness balance experimental paradigm.

Primary Auditory Beats The psychological perception experienced when two pure tones of slightly different frequencies are mixed and presented monaurally to a listener. The perception is that of a tone waxing and waning in loudness over time.

Propagation Velocity The speed with which a disturbance moves through a medium.

Psychometric Function The relationship between levels of a physical stimulus and the responses of an observer who has to make judgments regarding certain perceptions of the stimulus. When plotted, the psychometric function usually resembles a sigmoid function with the percentage of correct responses, or a specified judgment, displayed on the ordinate and the physical parameter of the stimulus on the abscissa.

Pure Tones Sounds characterized by spectral energy at a single frequency. Pure tones are sine waves we can hear.

R

Rarefaction During the propagation of a sound wave, regions of lower molecular density or pressure, compared to equilibrium.

Ratio In mathematics, a quantity that represents a proportional relationship of one quantity with respect to another. In the case of the decibel, which is based on a ratio relationship between two sound intensities or two sound pressures, ratios are unitless when they relate to quantities of the same dimension.

Ratio Scale A type of numbering system or scale in which the numbers representing the scale are proportional. A ratio scale also implies that mathematical operations, such as multiplication and division, are meaningful, and there is a true zero.

Recognition In experimental psychology, the awareness that a perceived stimulus is familiar and identifiable. This is the third level in the hierarchy of auditory behavior.

Recovery Interval In the experimental paradigm used to measure long-term poststimulatory auditory fatigue, the silent interval between the offset of the fatiguing stimulus and the onset of the signal for threshold measurement in the experimental condition.

Rejection Rate A quantitative measure of the slope of the skirt of a filter. The unit is typically dB/octave (decibels per octave).

Release from Masking The improvement in auditory sensitivity when both ears are allowed to participate in a noisy listening condition.

Repetitive Linear Motion The most fundamental kind of vibration, characterized by an object's moving back and forth between two extremes regularly over time.

Resolving Power A measure of the relative discrimination sensitivity of an observer.

S

Saturation The point at which the presentation level of a stimulus is high enough to drive the neurological activity of the neural fibers of the auditory nerve to their maximum level.

Sensation Level (dB SL) A type of reference for the decibel based on the lowest sound level that an individual listener is able to detect for a particular type of signal.

Signal In masking, the stimulus that the listener is trying to detect.

Simple Harmonic Motion A type of repetitive motion that forms the basic building blocks of more complex vibrations, including certain kinds of sounds. The motion is periodic because it repeats itself regularly over time and is defined mathematically as the linear projection of uniform angular velocity.

Simultaneous Dichotic Loudness Balance The name of the experimental paradigm used by Thwing (1955) in his investigation into loudness adaptation. The paradigm involves a loudness balance procedure, although it is more complicated than usual because both ears are presented with stimuli at the same time.

Sine Wave An *x-y* plot of displacement, or amplitude, as a function of time of an object vibrating with simple harmonic motion.

Sone A unit of loudness obtained using a direct procedure of loudness estimation. One sone is equivalent to the loudness of a 1,000-Hz tone presented 40 dB above the listener's threshold at 1,000 Hz.

Sound Field Conditions characterized by sound delivery from an external source some distance away from the listener. Sound field contrasts with signal delivery using headphones.

Sound Pressure Level Reference (dB SPL) A common reference for the decibel that is based on the physical pressure of a sound. The reference is .0002 dynes/cm² or 20 μPa.

Spectrum In acoustics, the two-dimensional display of a sound's amplitude as a function of frequency. The plural form of spectrum is spectra.

Starting Phase The relative position of a sine wave when oscillation begins.

Stimulatory Phase The second of three stages of a simultaneous dichotic loudness balance experimental paradigm.

Stimulus Duration The length of time that a sound is presented to a listener.

Summation The result of the combination of two sine waves that are identical in amplitude, frequency, and phase. A new sine wave sharing the same frequency and phase of the two component sine waves results, but the amplitude is the simple sum of the constituent waves.

T

Temporal Integration The ability of the auditory system to trade the effects of stimulus duration and stimulus intensity, for sounds characterized by short durations, in order to maintain audibility.

Temporary Threshold Shift (TTS) In the experimental paradigm used to measure long-term poststimulatory auditory fatigue, the difference between the thresholds of the signal in the control condition and the experimental condition. TTS is measured in terms of the decibel.

Threshold in Quiet In masking, the absolute threshold of the signal when presented in the absence of the masker.

Threshold of Audibility Typically, the experimental evidence from Sivian and White (1933). These thresholds represent the lowest limits of normal human auditory sensitivity across the audible frequency range.

Time-Intensity Trade The symbiotic relationship between stimulus intensity and stimulus duration for relatively brief sound in order to maintain audibility. *See also* Temporal Integration.

Tonotopic Organization A theory of frequency organization at several levels of the auditory system. This theory refers to the fact that pure tones close to each other in frequency are represented in topologically neighboring places at the level of the basilar membrane and beyond.

Transient Sound A type of aperiodic sound characterized by a very short duration.

Transverse Wave Motion A type of wave motion in which the particles of the medium move perpendicularly to the propagation of the disturbance. Water waves exhibit this type of wave motion.

Tuning The relative ability of the ear to perceive differences in stimulus frequency.

Tuning Fork A simple, metal, two-pronged fork with the tines formed from a U-shaped bar of steel. When struck, the tines of the tuning fork vibrate with simple harmonic motion to produce a pure tone.

U

Uniform Angular Velocity In simple harmonic motion, the characteristic of an object moving in a circle at a constant speed.

Upward Spread of Masking A highlight of the asymmetry of masking by a pure tone where the effectiveness of a frequency-restricted masker is greater for pure tone signals with frequencies higher than the spectral frequency of the masker and less for pure tone signals with frequencies lower than the spectral energy of the masker.

V

Velocity In physics, the rate of change of position of an object in motion. The unit of velocity is distance over time. Velocity is similar to speed.

Vibration The mechanical movement of an object, over time, around a central point or equilibrium.

Volley Theory/Rate Theory of Pitch Perception An important theory of pitch perception first suggested by August Seebeck in 1841. The fundamental premise is that the pitch assigned to a particular sound relates primarily to the temporal characteristics of the neurological impulses generated by the single fiber neurons innervating the length of the cochlea.

W

Waveform In acoustics, the two-dimensional display of a sound's amplitude as a function of time.

Wavelength In the propagation of a sound wave, the distance covered by one complete cycle of disturbance in a medium.

Weber's Fraction In experimental psychology, the expression $\Delta S/S$.

Weber's Law. In experimental psychology, a theory proposed by Gustav Theodor Fechner postulating that differential thresholds of sensitivity are related by a constant proportion of the original stimulus magnitude. Mathematically, the theory is expressed by the equation $\Delta S/S = \text{constant}$

Wideband Noise A complex aperiodic stimulus characterized by a continuous spectrum that is constant in amplitude throughout the audible frequency range.

X

x-y Plot A two-dimensional display of the effect that different levels of an independent variable has on a dependent variable.

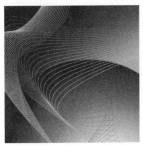

INDEX

Note: Page numbers in italic type indicate material in figures or tables.